Big Changes from a Small Stomach:

A Nurse's Transformation After Weight-Loss Surgery

Rachel L. West, PhD(c), RN

ISBN: 0692690875
ISBN-13: 9780692690871
Library of Congress Control Number: 2016907748
LCCN Imprint Name: **Driftwood Wellness Group, Lynn,
MA**

Dedication

This book is dedicated to my treasured "sleeve"
family and to every person who has ever stared down
(and lost) the battle with an Oreo.

Preface

According to the National Institutes of

Health, 68.8 percent of adults in the United States are

considered overweight or obese. It seems like

discussions about healthy living, mindfulness, and

weight reduction are everywhere. One need only scan

television and the Internet to see the effect of the

multi-million-dollar diet industry.

For so long advertisers have thrust into our

consciousness the undesirability of being overweight.

Of course, as a registered nurse, I can tell you

firsthand about the detrimental effects of obesity on

the human body. But that is not the intent of this book.

This book is not a manual for how to "lose

Rachel West

*weight" or "be mindful," though you will learn tools
and techniques through my stories that might help you
on your journey of self-discovery and self-love. This
book is not aimed at admonishing the diet industry or
the processed food industry, though you will learn,
through reading, the flaws these two industries exploit
to profit off our individual and collective suffering.*

*You will find contained herein a description
of the process I have gone through as I have come to
find out who I am. Some of the realizations I have
discovered have startled me, some have brought joy,
and others sadness.*

*I realized through conversations with other
bariatric patients that my story might help provide
direction and insight into the lessons we need to learn
to lead full and productive lives. While every obese
patient travels an individual journey, there are*

similarities in all of our stories. There are lessons we all need to learn about being reflective, thoughtful, and forgiving as we engage in behaviors that will help us develop our true and positive selves.

This book has been a labor of love. I have poured into it my joy, sadness, weakness, and strength. The process of becoming a bariatric patient is unique to each individual and this is my story. I attempt to describe the circumstances and experiences of what led me to become a bariatric patient, the experiences in the immediate pre- and postoperative phases, and the lessons I have learned as I continue to travel on this journey. The information presented in this book is as accurate a description as my mind will allow.

The people I have described in this book are based on people I have met along the way. Their stories have been included with their permission. My goal—and I hope that I have succeeded—was to sketch their nuanced personalities and attributes fairly. Some names may have been changed.

1 The Middle

Leaving work at an unheard-of hour to make
it up Coors Boulevard in Albuquerque to meet him, I
was nervous. I hadn't told my coworkers where I was
going or what I was doing. I wanted this to be my
private experience. "A doctor's appointment," I gave
as my reason for needing the afternoon off. As I
walked toward the big beige stucco building, the wind
whipped outside. The winds were always strong in the
early spring.

Sometimes, as was the case that day, the wind was so strong the dirt landscape would whip up and sting my face. I was early for the appointment, which meant I would have to wait in the waiting room. After all, doctors are never on time. Between the pelting dirt on my face and the leaps in my belly, I was amazed at my forward trajectory across the parking lot.

The slow automatic doors opened, and I walked inside. Two elderly volunteers sat at the information desk wearing royal-blue smocks. They asked if I needed directions. "No, thank you," I replied. I knew where I was going; at least I thought I did. In reality, I had no idea where this appointment would really take me.

The relatively empty open spaces were neat and clean. The big, bright floor-to-ceiling windows showed the windstorm outside blowing around sand

and the debris of the city. I was happy to be inside, at least for a moment. The slate floor struck me as unusual for the space; it made the seating area feel more like a living room and less like what it really was. The space did not at all feel like a hospital.

I regretted wearing my heels that day, as there would be no way I was sneaking up on anyone with the click-click of each footstep. I turned the corner and continued walking away from the dust storm. The office was at the end of what seemed like an eternally long hallway. "BARIATRICS," the sign said, making sure that anyone who was there would see that I was headed to the "BARIATRICS" department. Despite my conscious mind telling me this appointment was a fool's errand, that I wasn't that overweight, my grandmother's words pierced my thoughts, and I walked on.

Her last coherent words to me before she died just a few months before were, "You have to do something about your weight." So there I was, walking toward an appointment that would literally and figuratively change my entire life. In the moment, I felt lucky that this little hospital had few visitors or staff, and I made it down the hall to the doctor's office unseen.

2 Waiting

There is something fantastic about feeling as if you have not been seen doing something that you would rather remain private. Perhaps this was a small victory in the moment, but my life was about to shift so completely—in every possible way that can be imagined—that the victory might have been short-lived. The waiting room was mercifully empty. The standard doctor's office sliding glass receptionist window was propped open and behind the glass sat a thin, blond woman with a warm smile.

"Hello, I have an appointment," I said.

"OK, fill out these forms and bring them back to me with your insurance card and ID, please," she said.

When I turned around, clipboard in hand, I saw the small waiting room—still empty. Another victory! The chairs were maroon and basically unremarkable. Some looked like average chairs; ones I would have, for sure, avoided in the past and now made note to avoid.

There would be significant time and weight loss before I would feel comfortable picking any seat. In fact, the first time I flew on an airplane post-op, the feeling of worry that I felt as I sat down—and that quickly evaporated once I was able to buckle the seatbelt with ease—caused so much joy I took a picture and sent it to everyone I knew! Even now, I still have a short moment of hesitation before I get on a plane (especially when I'm in the dreaded middle seat), worried that I will spill over to the other seats. I do not spill over to other seats anymore, and every time I fly now, I have the positive reminder that I am no longer that person, so I can get past that fear a little bit more.

Other chairs in the waiting area looked more like a chair and a half. Of course they had those chairs. I imagine most of their patients couldn't fit in an average chair. Who was I kidding? *I* couldn't fit in an average chair at that time.

The number of times an overweight or obese person considers situations like what kind of chair to use, or whether to go through the turnstiles at the movies, or sits on a couch and wonders, "Will I be able to get up?" is innumerable.

The striking reality is that there are so many moments in an obese person's life where self-imposed limits are set: I can't do (fill in the blank) because I won't fit/will look fat/will hurt too much/et cetera. Naturally, there are actual real-life, experiences that have led us to these limits.

For example, I wanted to buy a kayak a number of years ago. I pulled up to the store in a little sleepy town in Maine where I was vacationing. The boats were on the sidewalk in front of the store. The salesman, looking me up and down, suggested the biggest boat they carried. Yes, I noticed that change in the salesman's affect and his obvious assessment of my body shape. I had to get in the boat to "test it out" on the sidewalk, and as I did, the salesman watched unapologetically as I tried to fit in the boat. I made it part of the way. Getting out was less than graceful.

The insult to my pride and the supreme loss of confidence of that experience still pulls at my ego some today when I remember the incident. Now, multiply this incident by a million similarly small but profound experiences, and it is no wonder that the root of obesity lies in the painful emotional baggage we carry around. One very important lesson I have learned in this journey to date is that while the past influences our present, it does not control our present and absolutely does not control the future.

I took the clipboard and the pen, which had taped to it a large plastic gerbera daisy, and made my way to one of the extra-wide chairs. The hospital's logo was gerbera daisies. Sometime later, I wondered if they chose daisies because of the way people view them. They represent fresh new beginnings to many people. I felt a degree of comfort having that happy flower bob along with the motions of the pen as I wrote deliberately on the intake forms.

As a nurse, I am conscious about how I write on forms because I know other professionals will interpret and read them. I was careful with my replies to questions about my past medical history and current weight-related complaints. Nothing was false, of course, but I felt it was important to be careful about how I answered the questions. In other words, I felt I needed a filter.

I completed the forms and returned them to the woman behind the glass. The butterflies in my stomach, which were there before, were starting to flutter even faster now. Was this really happening? Was I really in the waiting room of a bariatric surgeon?

Despite trying very hard to appear calm, I'm

sure I must have looked terrified. A shorter woman appeared. Not thin, but not terribly overweight, either, she had short dark hair and a warm smile. She introduced herself as Jeanne, and we began to talk. We talked about nothing terribly important—the weather, the season, and so on. She made the brief wait much more bearable, like a merciful angel there to help me pass the time. She was funny, and conversation flowed easily.

Before long, it was time for my appointment. I have always thought I was particularly observant— seeing details, noticing nuances that others never notice. Now I can see the irony in the lack of skill I possessed of noticing nuance in myself. I was in serious denial at my size and general unhealthy state of being. I still shudder when I look back at old pictures.

In reality, the hyper vigilance I kept to be aware of my surroundings came from what I now know to be fear. Being overly observant had become a safety mechanism in order to completely understand my surroundings; I could make barriers and try to fit in or disappear. Now, more comfortable in my skin, I am able to trust myself more and limit the urge to try to control situations that I know I cannot control.

It was time. I had to be weighed, measured, and evaluated. I followed the tech through the double doors to the back hallway. Off to the left was a very wide scale. The scale looked industrial. A sense of loathing bubbled inside me. Begrudgingly, I stepped on the scale. The red numbers flickered and read: 296 pounds.

No, that couldn't be. There must be a mistake. I had little reference, as scales were not allowed in my house, but this seemed unreasonable. The last time I was weighed was at my obstetrician's office two years prior after delivering my third baby. Literally, I requested that the tech weigh me again. She smiled a knowing smile. This time it was 297 pounds.

"No more weights!" the little voice inside me screamed, and then I shrunk in shame. I began one of the internal dialogues that now I recognize as harmful and hurtful.

"How could you let it get like this, Rachel?" I thought. "Oh my gosh, you are almost three hundred pounds! Don't you have self-control? Why can't you get this figured out? Oh my gosh, are you really thinking surgery will cure you? What are you thinking?" the thought train raged on in my mind. I tried to shake those thoughts out of my mind and did, to some extent in the moment.

One of the first steps an obese person must take is to release the negative feelings we attach to inanimate objects—like the scale. After all, the scale didn't do anything to me but tell me a number; a number I now know only tells the physical weight of my body, nothing else.

The number on the scale does not describe my sense of humor, my wit, my intelligence, my successes or my failures. In fact, neither does the size of my pants or the section of the store I shop in tell me about my worth as a human being yet we give these things inordinate amount of power over us!

Finally, we made it to the exam room. By now I was feeling rather anxious. The nursing assistant took out the extra-large blood pressure cuff and measured my blood pressure. It was no wonder my blood pressure reading was slightly elevated as I tried to regain focus and calm down.

I remember wondering in that moment how much longer it would be until I could use the "regular" adult-size blood pressure cuff. I've graduated down a size now, and that feels good! Each small victory, like the size of the blood pressure cuff needing to be smaller, only adds to the overall feeling of success and personal worth I have now.

I doubt very much that most people would consider the size of the blood pressure cuff or what that meant about their worth, but I did. I, like many people, assign a large amount of importance on being the right size, average size, normal size, healthy size. Being abnormal by using the extra-large (sometimes called "thigh") cuff was another small, but powerful, reminder that I was unhealthy, overweight, and bigger than I thought I was.

We are all subject to the trappings of the media and advertising showing us images of unnaturally thin models with unnaturally super smooth skin to encourage us to buy whatever it is that the company is trying to sell. Unfortunately, after repeated exposure, we no longer see the item for sale, but rather the image of the way we are *supposed* to look.

Next, it was picture time. She had a camera. Yes, there would be pictures. I have never seen the photos, and I am sure I never want to. The person in those photographs is now dead. She is gone, forever.

After the photos, the tech asked me the usual questions and left me alone to sit in a gigantic chair I decided it was designed to accommodate the ultra-morbidly obese. I purposefully sat squished to one side. I thought if I sat so that anyone who came in could see I was taking up only a small part of the chair, perhaps the person would maybe respect me more. I recall feeling, in that moment, quite embarrassed that I would inevitably have to tell the doctor I was a nurse.

I dread the exam room conversation whenever I am at the doctor's office for any reason; in *this* office, the feeling of dread was the same or maybe slightly worse. I loathe the feeling of having to explain my symptoms, my issue, my concern—and then ask questions, and seek clarifications like I have no idea what is going on and need help. I don't like to ask for help or to seem weak. I am the caregiver, not the care recipient.

My mind was a flurry of activity. The butterflies had turned to knots. Nausea crept in, and I desperately wanted to leave. I nervously scanned the room, looking at the awards on the wall, the anatomical models showing the lap band, and a nutrition chart describing the vitamins and other nutrients needed to be healthy.

There was a large and otherwise unremarkable desk, a comfy-looking office chair, and a small exam table. The exam room was enormous compared to any other exam room I had ever been in. I felt as though it would swallow me whole. In fact, it may have if it took any longer for him to arrive. My eyes settled on the extra-wide door.

"Maybe I should leave," I thought.

When I heard something at the door, I brought my hands to the armrests and began to shift my weight. I paused, stuck in the moment. My breath again stopped, waiting...

3 Dr. V

I heard footsteps outside, the distinct shuffle of the paper chart from the wall rack, and a pause. The door handle moved, and the door popped open. I lost my breath in that moment. I had goose bumps and a chill that I couldn't shake. My heart pounded so hard I could feel the hair on my head pulsing. He was looking at my chart—reading it. The door opened, and he walked confidently into the space.

Once I got the nerve to look up at him, I noticed he seemed to be swimming in his suit. I was not able to look at him for a while. Actually, in that moment, I was quite certain I would shatter into a million pieces if I looked too closely at him. I shifted my gaze elsewhere and tried to remember to breathe once again.

He moved, with purpose, directly toward me. I was sure I was about to pass out. Thankfully, at the last moment, when the room began to sway, I remembered to breathe. He plopped in the chair with little thought and turned to face me. I could feel his eyes burn a hole through my body.

I looked all around, while trying to look at him—or at least in his general direction so as not to seem rude. I saw his short black spiky hair swirling up to the top of his head, the way the suit jacket sat on his shoulders. I was uncomfortable to say the least, but I knew that I must tame my inner nerves and summon something that resembles order on the outside.

I drew on my professional skill set. Many times I had found myself in situations that other people would find uncomfortable—telling a son that his mother died before he could get to her to the hospital or discussing cessation of treatment of cancer and the initiation of hospice care for an otherwise healthy-appearing forty-six-year-old father of three young children. I've had to discuss with students the inevitable reality that they will not complete the semester with passing grades, and sometimes that means dismissal from the school of nursing, dashing their dreams of becoming a nurse.

I can handle difficult conversations, when they aren't about me. I'm sure Dr. V would have something insightful to say about that phenomenon, and someday I might get the opportunity to ask him. I somehow found the strength to breathe again and decided that I could, I would, look at him.

When I did, I looked in his eyes. He was watching me. I was sure in that moment he was aware of my discomfort. Over the years of knowing him, I have come to know that he is a very intuitive person, able to know a lot about the world just by being in it, open to the messages that the universe is sending. His eyes are dark pools framed in a soft almond shape. The faint lines around his eyes reveal that he has smiled a lot in his not-so-long lifetime, but there is also sadness in his eyes.

My impression, in that moment, was that he suffers with his patients, and that he carries his own lifetime of sadness with him. I thought that his full investment in the task must increase the possibility of his being caught up in the stories of his patients. I know, as a bedside nurse in the intensive care unit, I would bring home my work, my patients' stories. The stories, good and bad, helped shape me into the nurse I am today.

Despite the sadness in his eyes, there is a spark, an energy in him, that shines through. Right then, the energy was focused on me. He has looked at each of his patients, I am sure, with the same sincerity and intention, and I am quite certain that even those patients who are only mildly self-aware have felt as I did: exposed, scared, and alone in that giant chair.

Of course, the feelings of fear quickly turn once he started to speak. His smile was real. He made lingering eye contact and paused to hear me speak. He seemed to want to hear what I had to say. With each question he asked, I simultaneously felt better and worse. I felt better because I was able to do something besides sit there as an absolute wreck, and worse because I was sure he thought I was a blundering idiot. I was sure I had not yet said anything of real value or answered any of his questions with any sort of clarity—I was much too self-absorbed in the moment.

Dr. V explained the surgical procedure and asked me many questions. He paused to wait for me to answer him. I could feel the tears coming with a line of questions in the middle of the appointment. He was asking me about my past life. What was it like growing up? Was I always obese? How do I feel about food? What are my favorites? I tried to answer.

I saw something change in his affect as he asked me these questions. He knew I was on the verge, and yet he pushed on. I described how beautiful, peaceful, happy, and wonderful my childhood was. I was not abused; I was not hurt. I was so incredibly thankful for that part of my history. I tried to draw on the lessons my grandma taught me, but he knew. He knew there was more to tell, and so he pressed all the buttons on my inner psyche until I came undone.

4 Truth

I positioned myself in that extra-large pink
pleather chair, so careful to appear at my greatest
advantage and yet, when I talked about my
relationship with food, I became a disheveled mess.
At first, the tears welled, then they spilled, and then I
was crying. Really crying. I was sure I was not
making any sense. It was as though a flood gate was
opened, and I was sure I couldn't stop. Dr. V sat with
me, and he softened. Thankfully, there was a
conveniently placed box of tissues on the desk in easy

reach. Obviously, tears were common for people sitting in that seat, a fact that made me feel both comforted and uncomfortable.

How did this happen? How did I let myself come apart like that? I practiced answers to questions that I imagined he would ask. I imagined what my answers would be to the inevitable questions about why I wanted this surgery or how I might handle the inevitable recovery challenges (despite the fact that I really had no idea!).

What I failed completely to imagine was how this surgery, this experience, would change every aspect of my life. Even though the realization that everything would be different was only the beginning glimmer of a thought in his office, I knew in those moments my whole life would change—and it has.

Beginning to realize that everything would be

different was scary and exciting. After reflecting

many times about my tears in his office that day, I

know that they came from shame. What was it that

brought me to such a state of discomfort and shame?

He was talking that afternoon about how perfect

babies are when they are born.

I had three children at the time, and I

remember their births and the subsequent love affair I

had with each of them. He talked about how we are

all perfect. In that pleather chair, wearing my

snazziest suit, and holding my sopping-wet ball of

tissues, I just couldn't see how perfect the moment

was.

It has taken me a long time—and a lot of

reflection and introspection—to assimilate the idea

that we are all perfect and that "all of us" means me

too. The shame comes from the feeling that I had

abandoned myself, that I let go of who I really am to become a hurt shell of a person. The accumulation of painful moments and a deficiency in self-love allowed me to become numb to the world and try to feed my pain with whatever I could find to consume.

He was firm, direct, understanding, and loving as he asked the questions, and I feebly replied. How can a person emit such sincerity and concern after what he has read in a chart and seen in a heap of blubbering mess? His words echoed the teachings I had heard and been subject to my entire life. It was as if my grandma Claire was right there.

In the moment, despite the flurry of emotions, I heard her as if she were talking through him. I heard her talking about loving ourselves, being patient with who we are, and being present and mindful. I heard her talk about the power of food—or the lack thereof.

"Can an Oreo really control you?" he asked pointedly and followed quickly with, "We are the most intelligent forms that we know of on this planet. We can build ships that take people to outer space, and we can't control ourselves with a package of Oreos? Of course we can," I heard him say impatiently, and his face changed from smile to frown.

His tone and manner of speaking were filled with passion and insistence. I believe this came from a place of confidence and a sincere belief in the truth of what he was saying. I have heard some patients say that this method of questioning is off-putting, and there was something very striking about it in the office that day. What I understand now though is that, while unique, the desired effect of peeling back the layers of denial we have laid over our true selves is an absolutely essential component of the program and lasting success at weight release.

Of course, he was right about the completely ridiculous notion that Oreo cookies could control me. And of course, in my rational mind, I have known the truth of that sentiment, too. Yet, despite knowing this truth, I again felt shame as I remembered that I had rendered myself utterly helpless when staring down an Oreo.

Eventually, as the tears ebbed, we got to the part of the appointment where he would do the physical exam. The sadness was immediately gone from the forefront of my mind, and dread filled the void. People did not touch me. Period.

Massages, for example, were a thing of the distant past. Despite many very stressful times in my life when a massage would have been helpful, I had denied myself that gift because I felt too large to be touched. I dreaded the feeling of the massage therapist's hands finding every lump and bump on my exposed body.

Denying myself a healing ritual that caused more pain because of the initial denial was an uncomfortable pattern I realized I was inflicting on myself. Once I knew the possibility existed for me to behave in such a negative way, I was much more aware of mitigating the risk to engage in that behavior.

Yet, here I was in the office, startled back to reality when I had to bear my squishy abdomen and endure inspection and evaluation. The rational mind was overpowered, and I was returned to the ball of nerves I had been only moments ago.

5 Clothes

The exam itself was basically unremarkable. I was glad that I remembered to put on nice panties that morning. I suppose this is another example of my need to please, to impress, and to try to exert some control on a situation where I cannot have any control. The more I travel along on the journey, the more I realize I have consistently tried to put up walls, build a façade, and filter my true self.

Of course, as any overweight person might tell you, if he or she could ever be honest about this subject, finding nice panties or nice clothes is somewhat of a fantasy. While there may be things we like to wear, they never really fit, and they are almost never the thing we really want to wear. We wear what we can find that sort of fits and then celebrate that "victory" despite the fact that settling for "sort of fits" or "doesn't look *that* bad" only further punishes our selves.

From what feels like being on the outside looking in, shopping for clothes and shoes for a large percentage of the population seems to be an activity of joy and anticipation. In the majority of the years of my young and early adulthood, the thought of shopping was intellectually exciting but in the moment it was upsetting, unsettling, and depressing.

There never seemed to be anything I could find to fit, let alone want to wear. For me, the biggest ill-fitting offenders were pants, and later, shoes. Pants were almost always wrong. The felt like they were cut for someone else; too big at the back of the waist, too tight at the hips, too short at the ankle. For years, I wished I could wear a belt to solve the gap at the back of the pants but, of course, no belt would fit, as they were all too short!

The disappointment of never finding shoes that fit is just too much to describe. Unless you have felt the disappointment of thwarted shoe shopping, you might never understand. Scanning the displays, looking for a not-too-pointy toe, a wide base, not too much heel, and then finding something that might just sort of fit and is not supremely ugly, and they don't have your size. Of course, they don't have the size. They never have the size!

Now, I understand the joy of shopping—of

imagining who I will be and what I will be doing when I wear that dress or those shoes. The idea is delightful, almost intoxicating. I get to *choose* what I *want* to look like.

I get to decide the image I want projected to the world, and I do not have to settle for whatever is baggy enough or hides that roll or covers *that* spot. When I shop now, I am imagining where I will be and what I will be doing when I buy that cute top or pants that seem to find and hold every curve just right.

As I develop consciousness and a willingness to learn about who I really am, I find that determining what my "style" is has been a bit more difficult. I am still a combination of contradictions. On the one hand, I am very happy to wear jeans, work boots, and a dirty old T-shirt and muck around in the horse barn. I love to garden and get dirty. I love the feeling of being "in" the dirt.

The therapeutic benefits of being connected with nature in a garden cannot be overstated. Knowing where our food comes from, and knowing that we have had a hand (literally) in tending and supporting the growth of that which will nourish us is a beautiful example of the circle of life. Americans have become so disconnected from our food. I was at the supermarket today and I heard a young boy, maybe thirteen years old, ask his adult caregiver to describe a cucumber, having never seen or tasted one.

On the other hand, I feel that since I know now much more keenly that we are judged by our outward appearance (and I am not injured by that assessment like I was for so many years), the clothes I put on to go to work or out to play with my friends, matters. Most importantly, they matter to *me*. I care what I look like, what I put out in the world. I care that I have combed my hair and wear clothes that fit well. I no longer try on ten outfits before selecting one because I wonder what others will see. Rather, I am now looking at the woman in the mirror, trying to determine if the way I look and the way I feel in what I am wearing is what *I* want.

I gravitate toward the classic look now. I am absolutely giddy when I can go into any store in the mall that I want and invariably find something that fits and then have to decide if I want to spend the money and take it home or (and this is the best part) leave it because I don't really like the way it looks!

I love dressing in fancy clothes and wearing panty hose. Panty hose no longer bring with them a sense of dread. I wear them now with relative frequency, showing the beautiful shape of my lower leg. Describing my leg (or any part of me for that matter) as beautiful is more evidence of the strong shift in my thinking and beliefs.

An interesting phenomenon that I have found continues to be an annoyance is the relative discrepancy in different manufacturers' sizing. I am a size 10 in one store and a size 14 in another. How is that even possible? Irrationally, I choose to shop in the stores where I am a size 10. I suppose full transcendence is fleeting. Perhaps the lesson is then, that some of the frustration I felt before was related to this inconsistency in sizing and not that which I told myself: I am unfit for the clothes in these stores; they couldn't possibly make those cute clothes for "someone like me."

Interestingly, shoe size is relatively stable. After the initial drop I experienced in shoe size at the beginning of the weight release, I am relatively stable and relatively confident that I can, for example, order shoes online and be satisfied with what comes. I can readily find shoes in stores that not only fit, but fit well and are what I *want* to wear. I am liberated!

So much of the journey after weight loss is rediscovering the self; learning who we are and learning to love that person. People say they don't know who they are as their size changes, as their outward appearance can no longer hide the inner person. "Safety fat" an old college friend called it, no longer protects us from the outside world. We are open and exposed. We must discover who we are and learn to love that person.

6 Worth It

Back in the examination room, Dr. V and I continued talking. We talked about what my goals were, how the program worked, what I would need to do, and what he and his staff would do. I got a copy of his book. On the back, there was a picture of him, only it really didn't look like him. He saw me looking at it, and as I do not have a so-called poker face, I must have scrunched my brows. He said, while apparently reading my mind, "My twin brother." We both smiled and returned to the happy, positive atmosphere that I knew he worked very hard to

41

cultivate.

When it was time to go, I was filled with a multitude of conflicting emotions. I felt at once empowered and scared, regretful and hopeful, happy and sad. Some of his questions were pointed and severe and forced me to look at places I had previously felt too scared or ashamed to think about. I was invigorated to begin to think about the possibility that I could reinvent my life; I could be whomever I wanted to be. I didn't have to be unhappy; I didn't have to be self-limiting, self-doubting, and scared. I could seize my existence and make the life I wanted, which I have done.

There were times in the interview when I felt uncomfortable hearing the question and providing an answer I was sure he did not agree with. I could tell he was frustrated at my situation, my answers, my ideas, and my beliefs about how and why I was at the place I was. Of course, the answers were very simple to him—he wasn't living this life, struggling the way I had for years. I am sure he had, at that point, heard the side-stepping answers a thousand times. Now I know that it is simple to choose something else, to decide that I am worth "it." Whether I can always remember that our lives are simple, and it is our own doing that they seem complex is another story.

By the time the extra-long appointment was over, and I was making my way back out to the car, the wind had died down some. The same two volunteers in their smocks were parked at the door with newspapers now and little white coffee cups. As I made my way back to the car, I thought about how the volunteers seemed to sense that I was not as anxious as I had been when I came in, and they smiled very warmly at my leaving. Maybe I was projecting.

I cried for a while in the car. So many feelings came bubbling up in that appointment—some I knew were there but that were buried deep, and some that were surprising. I sat and wondered if I was doing the right thing. Could I really be considering having weight-loss surgery?

I had traveled a long road to get to that parking lot; many years of doubt, limiting myself, thinking I wasn't good enough, worth enough. Just taking the time to think about how much I had limited my life made the tears come even harder. The release of some of that pain felt so good. I was left with a million questions that flew by at lightning speed, just out of reach of my conscious mind.

Every now and again, I catch a glimpse of

myself slipping back to self-doubt. I find myself making excuses or retreating to avoid the pain of the situation, and I wonder if this is a manifestation of old habits, if retreat is a normal and expected self-preservation mode, or if I really have not learned anything at all. Perhaps our biggest objective while on this journey is to remember that we have some tools to use, to lean on, when our old ways return; to send packing our negative feelings, without the use of food, and remember how special we really are.

The way that we individually check our thoughts and feelings and help them find their way back to an unclouded perspective is different. For me, I find that journaling, meditation, and positive rituals are very helpful. There are as many different manifestations of positive rituals as there are individual people in the world.

I know, for example, that the exercises I do every morning when I wake up are not making my body trimmer or thinner. Right now, the burpees and sit-ups are a ritual, an exercise in self-love that I do to maintain my current body shape status quo. When the demands on my time ebb, I am able to carve out time to run and swim.

There are times when all I have is my "floor work" in the morning right after meditation, and I remember to be grateful for the ability to move with relative ease and flexibility. I find I crave movement differently than I ever have in the past. I want to move my body. I feel strong and alive. I realize when I am moving and exercising that I am, without apology, worth the effort to feel good. I am worth it!

7 The Beginning

I can, from the earliest of times, remember feeling as though I was in a hurry. The urgency I felt about wanting to get out of my small town was intense. I never felt like I fit in. My parents, who did not feel that they fit in, shared a story and a truth that I adopted as my own. "Well, we aren't from here," they would say.

The school in New Hampshire was small; my class had twenty-three or twenty-four students.

Everyone in the class seemed to know one another. They went to pumpkin patch preschool and were friendly. I was from New York. This fact alone of being a "flatlander," as they called it, was enough to cast a shadow on me for a long time. In New England, perhaps the worst place you can be from is New York. Why? I'm not sure, but I bet it has something to do with the sports rivalries. Or maybe the issue is a long history of outsiders coming to conquer. In any case, at six years old, I felt quite out of place.

Thinking about my first day in second grade, I can still remember feeling nervous about what my new friends would be like. I was six years old, and I remember my parents telling me that they had to fight the school to allow me to be in second grade since the education I had on Long Island was good and my academic abilities would fit better with the second grade curriculum. I felt even more different and out of the norm.

As I walked into the only second grade classroom for the first time, I felt my face flush red. Why were they looking at me? Was I that different? Could they tell I was only six? Were my clothes OK? What are they thinking? I don't suppose I will ever know. I walked into the classroom, which was bright and otherwise seemed friendly. I found my seat and began the work of trying to disappear and simultaneously to excel in any way that I could.

Over the next several years in school in New Hampshire, I remember many occasions of feeling like I didn't fit in. Mostly, I recall developing the attitude that I differed in terms of my body shape and size from the others I went to school with. I developed a preoccupation with my looks. Along with that preoccupation came a negative internal dialogue that I still fight against today.

In my class there was a girl I will call Elaine who was overweight. No one liked her. She had a unique face—round with an upturned nose.

The girls talked about her (sometimes with little attempt at discretion), and the boys teased her. We all looked a little funny back then. What kid, as a preteen, doesn't look at least a little funny? To this day, I am ashamed that I wanted to participate in what I can only imagine was torture for her.

I don't recall ever getting what I imagined that I might from my relative proximity to the teasing. I certainly wasn't part of the "in" crowd. I do not remember actively harassing this person, but the mind can be selective. Additionally, and more importantly, by not standing up and protecting her, was I not just as culpable? Yes, of course the answer is yes. I was participating by being passive.

I remember feeling the conflict of wanting to participate, because I thought I would gain the respect of my peers, and knowing that what others were doing was not right. I remember seeing her round face once visibly cringe when one of the boys made a particularly unkind comment. In that moment, I vowed not to be part of the pain others were inflicting on her. We became sort of friends, and I solidified my place as outsider.

Because of the small size of the school, and the limited other experiences available in rural New Hampshire, the kids in my grade became really the only people I knew. As is the case in any group, smaller subgroups form as the group dynamics change. I wanted so badly to be part of the cool kids' group (which felt like the majority of the class, of course) and not surprisingly, I felt different and out.

Nothing I did seemed to matter. I know now that nothing I did mattered because on the inside, I was so afraid, and I was different. I felt I could see the games the other kids were playing, and I remember so vividly rejecting the necessity to play them.

The games were social experiments—trying to wear the right clothes, or say just the right thing to the right people at the right time, having a boyfriend, and so forth. I was not able to see that the resolve I used to avoid the games was getting me to a better place. Instead, I felt that because I was different and uninterested in playing the games, I was even more different and so became even more ashamed.

Bodysuits were the fashion and colored jeans. Yay 1980s! My mom, hopeless in terms of cutting-edge fashion, tried to help me get the clothes I thought in the moment would make the difference. She bought me a body suit and colored jeans. I wore them in an effort to fit in. I so desperately wanted to fit in.

My mother is the ultimate advocate for me. She is my steadiest friend and confidant. She committed to me everything she had. She helped shape who I am, for better or worse. As an adult though, I have accepted full responsibility for my actions, behaviors, traits, goals, successes, and the times I have faltered. As Dr. Gordon Livingston says in his book, "the statute of limitations on our past traumas has largely expired." We must commit to personal introspection and intentional acceptance of responsibility for our life situation.

I was not ever super thin. My well-meaning parents attributed my slightly squishy body shape to my Italian heritage. "You have the family backside," or "You are big boned," they would say. I believed them, of course; their statements were logical. There was a free resignation to accept that my situation was not my fault—that I was a little thicker than the other people in my grade. I continued, for years, ignoring reality and soothing that pain with food.

There was a miniscule amount of my body mass that made a mini muffin top when I wore the maroon body suit with my soft teal jeans. Looking at old pictures, I see that there was very little fat rolling over the top of my jeans, but I know in those moments in fourth grade, what was there felt like a lot.

In each of us, our mind is quite skilled at distorting memories. I remember standing in the bathroom at school one day looking in the mirror and

thinking, "You are fat; that's why no one likes you."
Just writing those words thirty years later hurts.

Not having the luxury or ability to step back
from the moment and have a wiser and maybe gentler
frame of reference, only made my internal body-
shaming dialogue more intense. The negative personal
narrative continued for years until it became a habit.
The habit then started to creep into other aspects of
my young life.

I liked the feeling of being on a softball or
soccer team and wasn't particularly good, but not bad
either. However, as a result of dwindling self-
confidence, I withdrew from active sports because I
could never be as good as Jean or Sandy or any other
imaginary version of myself I wanted to live up to. I
didn't see the truth, that there was no competition
with the outside world. The only struggle that really

matters is the one to be better than I was the day before.

I began to loathe gym class—something the gym teacher, Ms. Stone, seemed to know. At the time, I believed she tried to make it her personal mission to make me miserable. I became the victim.

The victim mentality is a pervasive default for many obese people. The role of the victim releases the individual from responsibility for the current state of being. Eventually, each one of us must decide to shift from victim mode and embrace our individual experience.

Now, with perspective and a more forgiving spirit, I'm sure the gym teacher had other things to do than want to make a sixth grader feel bad. Nevertheless, in the moments of gym class, instead of feeling I had the power to use my body and make it stronger and healthier, I could only see the faults of my body, my abilities, and my strength. I thought to myself, maybe I am not cut out for sports. But I am a social person; I like being with others.

I always loved to dance. Around this same time in childhood, I had seen and had fallen in love with the movie *Dirty Dancing*. The way the characters moved intrigued and excited me. I wanted hair like Jennifer Grey's, and I wanted to move like the other dancers in the film. I loved the way my body felt when I was dancing. Mom said the way they danced in the movie was jazz and signed me up for a class in our town.

I went for a while to the dance studio that occupied the front of the bottom floor of the dance teacher's house. After I started classes, I was soon looking at myself in the giant floor-to-ceiling mirrors that lined one wall of the studio. I could see how my thighs touched and how my belly poked out some in my leotard.

Again, I felt different from the other girls. I couldn't see that we all had bellies that poked out some, and everyone had a different shape. I could only see my faults—no attributes. I was practicing critically judging my appearance and myself. In practicing applying judgments, I then developed other safety mechanisms—avoidance, humor, and so forth.

I loved to dance, I still do, but it has been many years now since I have even entertained the idea of dancing. I stopped about two months into the jazz classes and never went back. The self-imposed pain of watching myself in the mirror was just too much to bear week after week.

I told my mom that I didn't want to and she,

for whatever reason, didn't protest. Every time we drove by the dance studio my heart rate quickened a little and I felt a sadness come over me. I became very skilled at keeping that hurt part of me to myself.

Now, years later, and after surgical intervention, I realize that I had become very adept at covering up the hurt places. I ignored my true self and in doing so, formed a lens through which I saw only a distorted reality.

The lens has come off, and I am finally seeing my true self. I am ready to start pursuit of my truest desires. Sometimes those desires are joyous and other times they are sad. I am not afraid of either, but when we are able to look truly at our situations and ourselves, the clarity of thought and decisions that come from that place are unquestionable and, while sometimes very painful, the decisions we make in truth are necessary and right.

8 Getting Ready

Part of the bariatric surgery program involves going to group sessions. Every patient must attend group. No excuses, no special treatment. Everyone goes. Period.

Groups were held in what felt like the middle of the afternoon and required that I tell my boss that I had this meeting I had to attend weekly, and so I would be leaving work early. Luckily I am a nursing professor and did not have classes on Wednesday afternoons. It struck me in the planning for the meetings that it felt like the universe was finally starting to work for me instead of against me. The victim mentality was shifting; I was able to choose a different perspective and it felt good!

My boss, the dean, whom I will call Tania, had the unique skill of generating a thoroughly penetrating gaze that created an on-the-spot feeling, which made me (and countless others) feel uncomfortable. Most of the time, her pointed gaze was set at someone else and she and I felt like we were on the same team. I was thankful that I was rarely the recipient of her intense gaze. Usually we are both attacking a work problem together. One of the things that makes our work so enjoyable is that we both find our jobs a labor of love. We work very well together, and that is something I am very grateful for.

I walked into her office and said, "I'm beginning a pre-op program for a sleeve gastrectomy." Using the medical terms helped me normalize the experience. I found myself standing in her stark office mildly defending my decision.

"Well, you see, the education program is so comprehensive, and I just don't want to spend the rest of my life like this. I want to be healthy for my kids," I rattled off quickly.

"Of course," she said. She was nothing if not succinct. She asked no further questions and offered no other explicit support.

Tania is, I imagine, supportive of my choice and a true professional. If she disagreed, she kept her disagreements to herself. We don't socialize at all outside of work, as we have next to nothing in common. She is supportive, and I was not teaching during the time I needed to be away, so there were no work-related conflicts.

With the little effort that the conversation took, permission had been granted, and I had cleared one more hurdle. I was on my way. It was as if now the train had started to roll out of the station. I could feel some of the emotional baggage start to lift off me. I was moving, for the first time maybe ever, toward something completely for myself.

It was Wednesday afternoon. I was sitting in my end-of-the-aisle cube, when I looked down and saw the time: 2:20 p.m. I had to leave, and I did not want to be late. I could feel the butterflies starting again. I was nervous, but excited and happy. It had only been a few weeks since my initial appointment when I crumbled into tears in the doctor's office.

I closed up my work and headed out. Luckily,

Tania wasn't in her office, so I could leave without a discussion and confirmation of where I was going. I was still a little more than a little embarrassed about what I was doing.

Sometimes I felt like having the surgery was taking the easy way out, or that I was admitting defeat—that somehow, by asking for this kind of help, I was not up for the job of tackling and conquering obesity on my own. From talking to other group participants, several of whom have become friends, the feeling of embarrassment is very common.

In fact, when talking to other patients from the clinic, I realize that so much of what drives our pain is a feeling of embarrassment or shame. It would take many more months before I was more comfortable with my choice—long after I had the surgery.

I walked out into the blistering hot sun of the desert and made my way to the car. Even in the winter, the sun is so warm. Despite living here in Albuquerque for a little more than a year, I was still struck by the severity of the weather. I climbed into my big SUV, took the sunshades out of the window, and made my way to Coors Boulevard. The traffic was intense that afternoon, which did not help my excitement or nervousness.

I was impatient and frustrated that I chose not to leave work a few minutes earlier. The congested roads and abundant traffic annoyed me. I had a moment of clarity, and I was sad when I realized how unkind I was behaving (even if no one could hear the grumpy road-dialogue I was having with the other motorists). Grandma Claire's near constant reminders to count our blessings came blasting into my consciousness.

I fought back the tears, remembering that she was gone and that I couldn't talk to her anymore. As much as I sometimes couldn't handle the intensity of our conversations, I missed them terribly. She would know just what to say in these moments to calm my nerves or offer some perspective on the "big picture" while staying true to the moment. I missed her in these moments so profoundly.

I engaged the Bluetooth and called my mom to try to help me take the focus off my nerves. She helped some. We talked about other things. I complained about the desert and the dryness. She complained about her work. She told me how much weight she was losing. She had the surgery six months before.

I happily admitted that I was inspired by her. She had lost a lot of weight—and so quickly. I could hear the excitement in her voice as she told me about having to shop for new clothes so often.

There is nothing like having to go shopping because you literally have nothing to wear that doesn't fall off your body and then getting to the store to realize that you can pick what you want, not what you can fit into! Each time I experience this feeling of freedom, I smile, knowing that I have crossed another hurdle.

I pulled my big blue truck into the parking lot and gathered up the book and binder required for the meeting. I had read Dr. V's book as prescribed—though I admit not all the way to the end on this first meeting day. I found the book easy to read, and I am encouraged and invigorated by his words. They echo my grandma Claire so much. She was always teaching, trying to help me find a better way.

Every time I think about her, my eyes still well with tears. I wondered what she would have thought about weight loss surgery as I walked along the sidewalk. Quickly, I determined she would be very against surgery.

As wise as she was, she was quite insecure herself and spent many years in fear and worry. She would not, I don't think, have seen the merits of a program like this. Her self-limiting behaviors, I see now, were so ingrained in her. I am not sure she would have believed that she was worth the risks of surgery, to put herself first, to be brave to look inward to find what made her truly happy and pursue it with the utmost vigor and passion.

One of the most important lessons I have

learned as I have lived during this time is that we must check in with ourselves. We must be aware of our feelings so that we can react to them in ways that are more constructive. Even now, years later, checking in with myself and making sure I am not inadvertently covering up my true self is an important ritual. I accomplish this with my daily meditation.

"Why would you want to cut into your body?" Grandma Claire would say, I bet. "You can do this. Meditate more! Become a more dedicated vegetarian! See a therapist! It's all in your head!" Of course she is right, I think to myself, rounding the bend in the sidewalk and marching onward toward the front of the hospital. She didn't know my mom had the procedure, but she knew that Mom lost a lot of weight. I know it made her very happy to see my mom getting healthier.

I admit that I feel a little sting at knowing that my grandma will never see me as I am today or as the person I am becoming as a result of the surgery. Maybe though, she always saw who I really was and that I was hiding in fear. Maybe it was because she really saw me and my potential that she pushed me so hard. Maybe the reason I always felt her words so keenly was that I too knew I was hiding.

9 Group

The group meetings were held in the same
waiting room I tried to sneak into a few weeks before.
Interestingly, the same two volunteers were at the
desk. I wiped the tears from my eyes as I walked
through the same slow automatic doors and made my
way around the open space to the long hallway.
Already the "BARIATRICS" sign seems less
daunting; in fact, it isn't quite as big as I remember it.
I hear many more voices, though it isn't loud. I pause
at the beginning of the long hallway to try to take it

all in.

For as long as I can remember, I have liked to pause and take in the scene before jumping in. I like to be an observer, I tell myself. I like to feel prepared—in control. I'm still learning to let go. I looked down the long hallway at the people milling about at the end. I was pulled from my thoughts by my perception that someone was behind me.

"Is this where the meetings are?" the woman behind me asked tentatively.

"Yes," I said.

Together, we walked toward the voices, each of us lost in our own thoughts. We were obviously both nervous. Somehow, I found my strength and began some small talk.

"Is this your first meeting?" I asked.

"Yes," she said, "you?"

"Yes," I replied.

"I'm Erin," she said.

"Hi, I'm Rachel," I replied.

We got to the waiting room, which was full of people. Obese people. At first, I found the scene a little alarming; there was a lot of body mass in this room! I did not feel a judgment. Instead, it occurred to me as I paused in the doorway, that I was among friends. I knew no one there (except Erin, whom I just met), but I instantly knew I was in a safe place. These people waiting for group had been where I was, and they had survived. I came to know that not only had they survived, they were thriving.

My new friend and I made our way to the back doorway where we would be weighed. Waiting behind the doors was Dr. V. He was wearing a suit, of course, and had a white checked shirt on underneath.

His shirt reminded me of graph paper. Every time I saw him wear that shirt afterward, it made me remember this first group meeting. I focused on the pattern of the shirt instead of the uncomfortable feeling hanging over me so heavily. I was aware that I again needed to remind myself to breathe.

I was startled to see him so actively engaged in the weighing-in process. I was immediately unnerved. What would my weight have done in the few weeks since I was here last? Will I have lost enough?

I was sure to keep a healthy distance between my new friend and myself as she went through the process of signing in and getting on the scale. I was careful to avert my eyes. Nobody likes the feeling of being watched while being weighed; not that this concept seemed to phase Dr. V!

My heart pounded as I signed in and took off my shoes. I could feel the doctor looking on behind me. I felt my face get red as I approached the scale, and I forced myself again to remember to breathe. I focused on the graph-paper shirt he was wearing to try to take my mind off the situation.

Even with the distraction, I was shaking a little as I got on the scale. I reminded myself again to draw on my personal skill set. I had helped resuscitate people who were barely clinging to life. I had witnessed miracles in joy and death, and yet the simple act of stepping on that scale made my body tremble. I was struck by the complexity of the emotions that surrounded being obese!

The results were in. I was down eight pounds.

Phew! I was smiling. The doctor was smiling. He called me by my name and congratulated me on my progress. It struck me that he knew my name. What kind of provider knows his patients' names and can recall them so easily? This was not a tiny practice, and I was struck by the personal connection he seemed to have with his patients.

Erin had left the scale area but had saved me a seat in the crowded waiting room where group would take place. I was thankful that we met in the hallway and happily sat down in the maroon chair beside her. We passed the time talking about the city, the desert, the weather, our families.

I was amazed and impressed that she had five kids. Wow! I thought I was busy with three. Erin did not seem overwhelmed at all. She had a sweet smile, and I enjoyed talking to her. A few minutes later, the doctor appeared, smiling widely, pushing the same big black office chair from the oversize exam room.

The group began. Group sessions are run the same way each time, I learned over the course of the next several months. Today though, it was my first group session. I was new and unsure of what would happen next. The desire to be a fly on the wall was strong as the idle chatter in the room dimmed and Dr. V started to speak.

"Hi, everyone," he said, quickly following with a perky "How is everybody doing?"

We all nodded and sort of muttered. There were about fifteen people in the waiting room. Some patients had had surgery some time ago, and some had had surgery just the day before. I was amazed at how well those fresh postoperative patients were doing! I gave them my thirty-second nursing assessment and decided they looked good! Some group members were having surgery in the next week or two, and then there were the newbies still at least a month out. The newbies were the in minority that day.

The program is growing, which makes me feel happy. I recognize the effect that this program has had on me, and I've only been a patient a short time. I am happy that many more people can be affected. I have come to appreciate the message of self-love and knowledge and the relationship of those two concepts to the foundation of substantive healing and growth.

There is work to be done in the group sessions. Work includes learning new foods and food preparation techniques and releasing fear to try new things. Other topics in group involve the more important work of changing attitudes, beliefs, values, and our individual internal dialogue.

Each group member finds challenge in the lessons differently. We are all walking along on connected, but separate, paths. Group members listen as Dr. V provides an overview of a topic, and a short question-and-answer session follows. An important part of the pre-op program is for participants to learn the fundamental three rules. New participants are called on to recite the three rules. Even to this day, those rules and those sessions still help guide me.

Obesity is an outward expression of internal suffering and so much of the work required is individual and psychological. Not until years after surgery do I even begin to feel the self-actualization aspect of this program coming into focus. In the beginning, group sessions were generally uncomfortable. I was not at all happy participating in the dynamic and difficult discussions in the moment, though I realize now how important they were.

Connecting with other people is a basic human need. We know that people who are isolated from other human contact develop behaviors that are, at best, undesirable. Connecting with other bariatric patients in the group setting helps the patient normalize the experience and offers a forum to validate internally held beliefs, attitudes, and behaviors. Now, via an online platform, we are able to keep connected and offer support and encouragement in the virtual world.

The support from those people has been incredibly valuable to me. Additionally, having a leader to guide the group who is fully engaged, passionate, and knowledgeable about the journey helps to solidify the lessons we are learning along the way. Over time, the constancy and presence of the members of the group help guide the way forward.

10 The Three Rules

Each group session starts with a review of the three fundamental rules of the program. New patients are put on the spot to demonstrate their mastery of the three rules. This practice is not done to alienate people, but to encourage meaningful connection with the challenging work surrounding the life transformation of bariatric surgery. Again, the personal connections we make with ourselves, the other group members, and the providers are what makes the program so dynamic, unique, and successful.

Each new patient is called on, by name, to say one of the three rules. Notes are not allowed. The rules and a discussion of them can be found in Dr. Vs book *Ultimate Gastric Sleeve Success*. I highly recommend this book, even if people are not considering bariatric surgery.

These rules guide the basic consumption principles for all of Dr. V's patients but they also speak to the larger philosophical umbrella that guides the program. We spend many weeks reviewing each point and the principles that guide each "rule."

One aspect of the program that speaks to my intellect is that Dr. V wants to teach his patients so that they can take the lessons to the world and be free of self-imposed burdens. The impact of these sessions cannot be overstated. A mid-nineteenth-century

British proverb is at the heart of the program: "Give a man a fish, he eats for a day. Teach a man to fish, and he eats for a lifetime." We are learning how to assess ourselves, how to nourish our mind, body, and spirit.

Take rule #1, for example. The rule states: lean protein first. The discussion that follows the introduction of this rule revolves around describing what a lean protein actually is. Lean proteins are things like beans, tofu, edamame, fish, and seafood. Gone are the days of grilled chicken breast! One of my favorite memories of early group sessions was where Dr. V was talking about no more boneless skinless chicken breast.

"Who eats grilled, boneless, skinless chicken breast?" he asked.

"Healthy people," someone answered.

"No," Dr. V said. "Who eats grilled, boneless, skinless chicken breast?" he repeated, smiling, knowing we likely would not guess his answer. A few more attempts at a reply popped out from the group. Finally, he gave up. We were a hopeless bunch, his expression seemed to say, but it seemed in the moment that his judgment came from a purer place.

"People on diets eat boneless skinless chicken breasts! People who are fat!" he exclaimed.

Hearing the word fat assaults my ears. It is a word I have never liked and like even less when a fit person says it to describe people like me. When I hear that word, I want to curl my ears in!

I remember the time in the bathroom from so many years ago when I first applied the label to myself each time I heard someone use the "fat" word. He expanded his explanation and in the process gave a very valuable lesson about why fruits and vegetables are the answers and why we should eliminate processed food from our bodies.

The second rule sparked a slightly more spiritual discussion. The essence of rule #2 is that our bodies are sacred and special. We deserve to have the very best. In fact, one of Dr. V's catchphrases is "You are worth it."

By owning the sentiment of being worthy of the very best, patients confront their own habituated self-loathing. As I have already described, the internal dialogue for many, if not all, obese patients is painful at times. For all the zillion reasons people have suffered, the internal negative narrative has been adopted and turned into a habit. The good news is that habits can be broken; we can learn a new way to react and think and in so doing can improve our mental health, which leads to better physical health.

Patients struggle most with acceptance of this rule. It means buying the better cut of meat (if they continue to choose meat—many people find a pescetarian existence much healthier and more in line with the teachings we learn). It also means treating the body to meaningful physical activity, purchasing a special new outfit to celebrate the new body shape, or generally just being more mindful to be respectful of our bodies. The personal work that surrounds successful integration of this rule in a lasting and meaningful way is something I still work on today, years later.

The third rule usually startles people. The third rule of the program is that we can actively choose to eat as many fresh fruits and vegetables as we can anytime we want. Why is this so difficult for people to believe? We spend so much of our time on "diets," limiting one food group or type. We focus on how many calories or fat grams a particular food has within. Instead, we are taught to buy foods without ingredient labels, to rely on the healthiest food we can find and buy to nourish our bodies. We are encouraged to try new fruits and vegetables to experience new flavors and explore the endless variations in cooking and preparation. We are challenged to expand our horizons and take the "I don't like that" sentiment out of our paradigm.

Since I have lived for a long time in this body and was even mildly aware of the food choices I was making, I felt annoyed and bothered that I would be taught how to eat; I arrogantly believed I had little to learn. Once I learned to let go of some of that fear and began to trust in the program and the teaching, I saw the successes mount.

The more I am able to let go of my incorrect assumption that I know all this already, the more successful I become. I am humbled and feel more than a little bit ashamed that I was so arrogant in the beginning. Of course, realizing this flaw allows some of the shroud to fall off my true self. I am able now to see more of who I really am and make different choices in the present moment and future moments.

A group member recently asked about how to begin to make the changes required by the program. Many people answered. Some said to make changes a little at a time; start with breakfast or focus on water consumption. Others said that the change has to be all at once.

It is my opinion that the change that has to happen must be all encompassing but it must happen in small and meaningful doses at an incremental pace with lots of forgiveness along the way. The changes that we will all face on this path are so great in number that to think about them would be overwhelming and off-putting. We must acknowledge that *everything* has to change and forgive ourselves because we are only human. We need time and space to fully integrate the teachings we are learning (or relearning), but over time we can and will make all the changes.

Trouble happens for patients when they stop thinking about the big picture, or they forget that they are worth "it." People I know who have had the surgery who have gained weight back and slipped into old habits, have done so because life got in the way and the focus on the big picture was blotted out temporarily. People I know who are most successful are those who do not take their eyes off the big

picture, or if they do, they quickly realize they have

stepped off track, *forgive* themselves, and get back on

the path to healthier and happier life.

11 Surgery

I heard the crickets of my phone alarm start their song. I quickly silenced the alert, quietly gathered my clothes, and got dressed. I had experience being up at this ridiculous hour, quietly getting ready, weekly for the last six months for the clinical rotation I was teaching in Santa Fe. I knew how to gather clothes and get dressed quickly and quietly. I glanced at the soft green glow of the alarm clock, which read 0518. I was right on schedule.

I made my way downstairs, gathered keys, and got to the car. It wasn't until I started the engine that I felt the first real wave of nerves. I was getting in the car, before the sun was up, to drive myself to the hospital to have bariatric surgery. As I considered this truth, tears started to well in my eyes.

I backed the car slowly out of the driveway and pointed the car in the direction of the hospital. I practiced positive self-narration as I made my way through the bright orange barrels that lined the road I traveled to get to the hospital. I was having this surgery to help myself get back the life I once had. I was doing this to show my children how to love oneself. I was having surgery so that I would not spend my adult life hidden under all this extra weight, which would, I was certain, lead to medical issues and poor health. I was doing this because I wanted to feel good again.

In truth, on that drive to the hospital, I struggled to find a time in my memory when I was last truly happy. I have had many happy times of course. The births of all my sweet and wonderful children are naturally at the top of my list.

With each delightful and joyous child brought more stress to an otherwise stress-filled life. I try very hard not to have regrets, but I regret feeling like I am not being emotionally present for my treasures as much as I could. I spent too much time worried about whether I was doing it *right* to relax and pour out love.

On that morning, as I made my way over the Rio Grande, I could feel my internal being starting to shift some, to give way, and open up to being a gentler person. I wanted to be kinder and gentler. I did not want to growl and be dissatisfied all the time, as I felt I had been lately. I wanted to remember to see the beauty in the world. There really is beauty in the desert as many have remarked before me. It has taken me a long time of living here among the shades of pink, brown, tan, and soft green to appreciate the simultaneous severity and softness of the landscape.

I pulled the car into the parking lot and walked toward the front door. The parking lot was empty and the air was crisp. No one was sitting at the desk. A phone sat on top of the counter with a sign to tell people like me to call for assistance. I picked up the receiver and told the person who answered what my name was and that I was reporting for surgery.

I made my way around the hallway toward the double doors of the OR suite where someone was waiting to escort me to the back. There is a certain amount of business involved in getting ready for surgery. Of course the business includes no clothes, a special bath with antimicrobial wipes, a swab of the nares with a truly horrible substance, answering a zillion times my name, date of birth, and what procedure I am having.

Being a nurse in this kind of situation is not actually comforting for me. I am much too aware of all of the potential complications, errors, hiccups, problems, and so on that are possible. I tried very hard to banish them from my mind as I prepared to get onto the stretcher and wait for my turn.

I noticed the clock: 0745. Jim, my now estranged husband, was due to arrive soon. He stayed behind to wait for the nanny to get to the house before coming to be with me. Of course, because of the self-imposed complexities of our lives and my desire to try to be strong, he would not be staying and waiting at the hospital for me much beyond my time in the recovery room.

I thought about my lectures on the intraoperative experience. I would have, for years to come, another wealth of stories to share with my nursing students to expand the classroom environment and make it more relatable.

I love teaching. I love being present in the moments where people are developing new skills, knowledge, and understanding. I love being there to help them shape their future nursing practice where they will undoubtedly care for thousands of patients in the best way that they can. I am proud to know that I am there with them on that journey, helping them to become excellent providers.

I realized as I watched the screen saver of

nature scenes on the TV monitor in the pre-op holding area and listened to the pleasant classical music, that that day was the day that I would mark when my life changed forever. I had made many of the mental adjustments that I could think of in the weeks leading up to the surgery.

The mental alterations I had made before surgery were nothing compared to what I had continued to experience long after surgery. Even in the moments right before surgery, I was aware of how little the surgical procedure drove the results. I knew that the true key to unlocking long-term success lay within me, my head, my mind, my actions, and my decisions.

Some of the mental changes I had made included things like how I was much more aware of what went into my body. For example, I could walk by the bakery in the supermarket and not feel the fear and dread of the doughnut case. I didn't need a special reward for making it through the grocery store, and if I did—the reward certainly wasn't food!

I had lived past that fear of not having cookies in the house—there to comfort me when I had a bad day. I remember walking through the grocery store on the day I decided not to bring the not-good-for-me stuff into the house. I remember a wave of fear that I somehow wouldn't have a tool I needed on the inevitable day that I felt I would need it. But I had worked very hard, and now I had some new skills.

Jim finally arrived, looking harried. It must have been a challenging morning, but I chose not to ask about it because I didn't really want to think about the possible drama. I was concentrating on having only positive thoughts that day.

The anesthesiologist came in, and I reminded him that the last time I had anesthesia, I had a wee bit too much (or maybe I am sensitive to it), so could we please take it easy. He assured me and hustled off. My next visitor popped in from around the side of the curtain. Dr. V had arrived. He seemed calm, which was good.

We discussed, one more time, what was about to happen to me, and I fought back tears. The doctor held my hand. I was comforted by this human pause. So often in the swirl of the US health care delivery system patients become dehumanized. Patients are referred to by room number, not name, and are barcoded and scanned. The refreshing return to the human state by the simple touch of a hand was refreshing and offered me one more ounce of validation that I was in the right place at the right time with the right provider.

I do not cry in front of people too often, though tears have always come relatively easily for me. My emotions are just always very close to the surface. My face will give me away *every time*.

In the little waiting area, wearing only the hospital gown and sheets, with Dr. V and Jim, I was vulnerable in the most real way I can imagine. I was going to be completely in the hands of others—open and unable to attempt to cover anything.

This moment was the beginning of the return to the real me, my truest self. A few minutes later, as the team wheeled me back to the OR on the stretcher, I remember feeling the hot tears roll out of my eyes as I cried silently. The tough outer shell I made to protect myself over the years had been cracked open and my true self began to shine through.

12 Post-Op

"Open your eyes, Rachel!" I heard a woman say loudly.

I tried and couldn't. I could hear her, though. I tried to speak. I am not sure if any sound came out. Two voices were there, one I recognized as giving a report. The first person, who must have been the post-op nurse, repeated herself several more times, but I literally could not move. I could hear what was going on around me. I heard her say that the surgery was all done, but I could not move, open my eyes, or speak.

I strained to listen to the report, to gather information about the surgery that would help me relax. Medicine, surgery, fluids, are all things I know about. I wanted so much to organize the experience, understand what had happened to me. I don't remember all that the two nurses reported, but I remember feeling satisfied when I didn't hear anything about too much blood lost or any obvious issues from the surgery.

The first voice of the receiving nurse kept at me with a raised voice, telling me to open my eyes and wake up. I felt like I was in a slow-motion movie because there were so many sounds and movements around the bed where I was, but I could see nothing and could not move. I knew that I needed to open my eyes, or she would never leave me alone, but I was so tired that I just could not do what she asked of me. I wanted to follow the directions and willed my eyes to open. They did not.

I could hear her voice changing toward impatient. "Come on, Rachel. Open your eyes. We need you to open your eyes."

I tried again and was able to open them somewhat, but just as soon as they were open, they slammed shut again. Eventually, I tried again to speak. With my eyes closed, I could make some words now.

"I'm trying," I said feebly.

Many more minutes passed, and I heard someone say that I was there for nearly two hours. Usually, patients do not stay in the post-op area very long—certainly not nearly two hours. It was time for me to go upstairs to the regular unit.

Once I arrived, I was able to open my eyes for short bursts of time but was not awake enough to hold a conversation or answer many questions. I understand that there are many demands placed on a nurse, as I am a nurse. I became somewhat unnerved though when my nurse for the evening was not sure what I was doing there or who I was. Perhaps, in retrospect, and with the dulling of memories that happens over time, the nurse was simply assessing my level of consciousness. Perhaps I will simply give the nurse the benefit of the doubt and believe that moving forward.

It was in those moments of faltering confidence in my caregivers, when I experienced truer fear than I think I had ever felt. Not only had I just had surgery, I was having some sort of reaction to anesthesia, and my night nurse was not confident in the reason I was on her unit. Jim had to go home to the kids, and I was to be left alone—unable to advocate for myself.

I realize that my experience is colored by the high expectations I have for myself and for society at large. I am aware that my profession, and experiences in health care, shape how I perceive the situation. I am aware that I was cared for adequately, and I survived. I made it to the morning and am here today, years later, able to write about my experience with little more than an afterthought about how it "could" have been. I am truly thankful for the relatively uneventful experience I had during my hospital stay.

The next morning the sun shone brightly through the window. I had a lovely view of the rooftop of another part of the hospital. The Sandia mountains are in the distance. I told myself to try to remember to look out on them in the evening to catch them turn pink, as they famously do every day. There was not much pain, and I could move around relatively easily. Mostly my midsection felt puffy and swollen.

As it turned out, maybe as a nice twist of fate, Erin was there on the same day, having her surgery too. We are now, as we like to call it, "sleeve sisters." We walked the halls together, past the well-meaning visitor who brought in three dozen doughnuts to the staff and left them on the nurses' station counter. We both chuckled at the well-meaning visitor and how much we appreciated that we would not, for the foreseeable future be ingesting anything found in a doughnut box.

I spent the next day or so in my room and

walking with my other sleeve family around the halls of the hospital, waiting to be released. There was no food, only ice chips and sips of water later in the day. I was feeling somewhat melancholy in the hospital. I was almost afraid to let myself feel happy about the change I had just made; like I was afraid if I wasn't careful it would all be for naught, and I would be somehow worse off for having had the surgery.

I did catch the mountains flare pink that evening. As I crawled into bed, I thought about my family, and I considered what having this surgery would mean for our relationship. I knew I was eager to have more energy and the ability to play with the kids. I wished I could talk to Grandma Claire and get her take on my current emotional health. She was always so good at cutting through the fluff and always knew the right thing to say (even if sometimes the right thing hurt a little to hear).

The next morning, I was served my juice-box formula drink and was told I could go as soon as I finished it. I was not in any particular hurry to leave but, not liking hospitals all that much, I did my best to get the thick vanilla-flavored liquid into me.

Midmorning, the doctor came up and met with the four of us who were getting ready to leave the hospital. He reviewed all the discharge instructions and answered our questions. There weren't really any significant questions, as the program is so education-focused it would be spectacularly difficult to get through the pre-op period, the surgery, and then get to discharge day and have many questions.

I spent several weeks at home, recovering and working to get my mind in the right space. I had restrictions on what weight I could lift, and I did get very tired. My hair didn't fall out too badly in the immediate postoperative period, thankfully.

I was so purposeful in moving around in the house, trying to manage the day-to-day responsibilities of caring for the three children and caring for myself. My mom came for a long weekend and helped some. I was so intently focused on getting my head around all that I had just been through. I recognized early in the process that the head is where most of the work is taking place for this procedure to have lasting and life-transforming effects.

I spent hours on the couch considering how I had let food dictate the bulk of my story. I had been conditioned to use food to comfort painful experiences and to further accentuate positive ones. As I took food out of the picture—because I literally

Rachel West

couldn't eat anything—I started to see the outside
world and experience it in a totally new way.

I started to see the immense beauty that the
desert has to offer, something I resisted for a long
time while living there. I started to see the
codependent rhythms of the wind and animals, the
requisite hardiness of the scrubby native landscape. I
saw with amazement, the severity of the weather.

When it is sunny, the sun shines so brightly
that it burns my fair skin very quickly. When it rains
(which it does very rarely), it rains so hard that
mudslides happen and flash floods are possible in the
otherwise bone-dry arroyo. The contradictions of the
weather are at once puzzling and beautiful.

I never noticed how the hummingbirds loved
my front tree the way I did in the immediate post-op
time I spent at home. I committed to buying a

hummingbird feeder and hung it out on the peach tree for them. I watched that feeder for the beautiful miniature green birds and saw them make a new habit of coming to have a drink in my front yard.

I gardened as I got the energy to do so. I trimmed the many rose bushes in the backyard and daydreamed about how to make the west-facing backyard more pleasant to be in for the family. I drew sketches of a backyard design to incorporate two large raised-bed gardens to grow our own food.

13 Food

After bariatric surgery, the physical space of
the stomach is smaller. No longer can we soothe our
pain, encourage our happiness, or calm our fears with
food. The searing pain, and associated cholinergic
responses (fast heart rate, sweating, dizziness, etc.) to
eating or drinking too much or too quickly will, for
the conscious person, deter future consumption in the
same manner.

One day, a few weeks after surgery (and

before I was back to work), I was preparing my go-to meal. I had a half an avocado, chopped Kalamata olives, and about ¼ tsp of crumbled feta cheese on a small plate. I had practiced eating slowly, taking small bites, and chewing food carefully to remember the texture and flavors of each morsel. On this day, though I was thinking about something else. I brought my mini lunch to the living room and sat down on the couch. Mindlessly, I ate the good food I had prepared. I ignored the subtle sign of "full," which for me is a hiccup. All it took was that one bite too many and nearly instantly knew I was in trouble.

I was home alone. I put the mini spoon down and sat straight up. My heart began to pound and sweat beads formed on my forehead. Pain stabbed my chest, and I was dizzy. I was breathing faster and feeling anxious. I wanted to cry, lie down, stand up, scream, be still, and move all at the same time. No position gave me relief. What had I done? Instinctively, as my mind was nowhere near rational at this moment, I raised my hands up over my head and began to walk around slowly. I tried to recall how to calm my nerves, as I knew that being anxious and feeling out of control would only exacerbate the physical feelings I was having. Thank goodness some of what I learned in nursing school came back to me in those moments.

Eventually, after what felt like an eternity, the symptoms began to pass, and I was able to catch my breath and bring my hands back to my sides. I looked out the window at the peach tree in the front yard and sat down. I looked at my mini bowl and my mini spoon resting on the cushion, and I vowed to myself that I would never let that happen again.

There have not, thankfully, been repeat events such as I had on that sunny day. I have never eaten so much that I had to vomit as some patients report. I am not perfect, though. I have, a few times, drunk water a little too quickly and felt a milder version of panic, pain, heart pounding to remind myself to slow down. Thankfully, with water, the pain and other symptoms dissipate quickly.

One of the greatest benefits of this surgery is being able to have a physical reminder of a psychological anomaly. While many people can gulp down their meals without incident (or tasting their food) it is much healthier to go slowly and be present in the moment. The physical hiccup, pain, or lightheadedness is the cue to remember that food is for sustaining life, not for curing ills, celebrating joys, or numbing pain.

Now, years past the initial surgical intervention, I can see some of the high and some of the low points with new clarity. The high points are easy to imagine—a new body, a shiny new perspective, a feeling of success and self-worth, which is likely unmatched in my individual history. Yet, the high points are just that: points. The euphoric feeling is so amazing and so warm, and it feels blissful. So, because life is about balance, and there cannot be light without dark, the high points dull.

Old habits creep back in, doubt and shame return to the mind. Almost without noticing that it is happening, we can find ourselves at a stalled-out place, a plateau. How many times in our dieting past have we heard or narrated things to ourselves, thoughts like, "Oh I'm on a plateau. I just can't seem to lose any more weight!" Well, the fact of the matter is that there are no plateaus. What has happened is that we have lost sight of the high points. We have forgotten to love ourselves first and to express that love in how we care for ourselves. The trick though, to not allowing a full and complete relapse/regain of weight released is to stop the mental boxing match, return to a gentler place of self-love, and start making new decisions.

We can find high places again when we remember to look for them. We have all the tools we need to find joy, peace, and happiness in our daily lives; we just have to use them! I recently read Helen Keller's piece from the early 1930s describing what it would be like for her to regain her sight for just three days. Ms. Keller's work described what she would try to see in each of the three days in an effort to capture the most important aspects of her human experience as an individual, part of a local community, as a member of the global community, and as part of nature. I am keenly aware of the necessity to go slow through the universe and really see what is here.

When we are moving too quickly and our highs become lows, we often describe this place as a depression. Depression is a manifestation of its close relative (let's call it a cousin) shame. Shame is, of course, a manifestation of fear, not love. Shame comes from one of two questions: "Am I good enough?" or "Who do you think you are?" So to "overcome depression," we have to understand which of the two questions is at the forefront of the current conflict and respond appropriately. The way to address the conflict is with the other emotion: love.

Of course some expressions of love for depression are: empathy, understanding, trust, and validation. I think my favorite way to express love to overcome depression is to count my blessings. When I can stop and see all the blessings I have and that I am, I am able to quiet (at least for a while) the "Who do you think you are?" question that so often plagues me.

I have tried to validate my personhood through the acquisition of degrees, titles, and distinctions that would otherwise set me apart from the pack. I realize now that the pursuit of those things is an attempt to answer the "Who do you think you are?" question. But are there other ways that I can find rest for that nagging question? Are there other things I can do to validate myself that would satisfy me?

Answers to these questions are still evolving and will, I imagine, do so for some time. One course of action that has been very helpful is writing this book.

The act of journaling is very helpful for many people.

I was never a teenager who kept a journal. In fact, it has only been a few months now that I have been keeping one. I never wanted to let my true voice out. I would censor my thoughts so that whoever might find and read the journal wouldn't get the *wrong idea* about what it was I was saying.

Now, after writing this book, I am very aware that many people will read my inner thoughts and will have varying opinions on what is contained herein. I know though, that many more will find what I have written, what I have shared—while scary for me to share—is helpful.

I have also started a consulting business that will help get this message, my story, out to the universe—to people who need to hear it. I strongly believe that health care providers must become more aware and more engaged with people in the preoperative and postoperative phases of surgical

weight loss. I still spend a great deal of time

considering my own growth and change. I still

practice a skill I first developed in my early

childhood, growing up in rural New Hampshire:

sometimes one needs to be still.

14 Stillness

After a long day at two jobs spread across the north shore of Boston, I would take the thirty-five minutes between when I got home and when I needed to leave again to snuggle with my babies before they went off to bed. The littlest one was ready for bed, but I managed to squeeze her before she headed to bed. The fuzzy heart-shape spattered romper she had on for bed only made her that much more snuggly.

I took mental snapshots of her chubby cheeks

and long, lean fingers as I fed her and put her to sleep. These mundane details would be the ones easily lost to the deep recesses of memory, but they are more meaningful than the richest treasure that exists anywhere. I remembered to keep the little moments close to my heart.

Miss L was my bigger focus tonight. She had been missing me the last few days (maybe weeks). We hadn't spent as much quality time as I thought we might have needed to, and so I took the few moments I had to love her up as much as I could. She got dressed for bed, and we read stories together on her bed. We snuggled, and then I was able leave with not one tear lost. I deliberately brushed the silky brown curls of hair off her face with my fingers, kissed her soft forehead, and slowly eased my way out of her room.

In these moments of clear focus, I was reminded of the importance of stillness. In silence we can hear our intuition. Whether we choose to listen to what intuition has to say is something else entirely. I was, just then, entirely in the moment of tucking Miss L and Miss M into bed. Being in the tender moments of letting the day go with my dear, sweet girls is truly the best gift I could have imagined.

Grandma Claire spoke a lot about being in the moment and the importance of being present. She would say to me, with relative frequency and definite urgency, "Be in the moment!" She knew I wasn't— she knew I needed reminding. Recalling these conversations, a wave of sadness washes over me as I feel regret for having taken so long to understand her message to me. What else have I set aside that I need to recall? What else do I need to tune in to hear?

Those questions have haunted me and have occupied a large part of my time in introspection. What else have I been consciously and unconsciously blinded from? Could it be that we truly don't know what we don't know?

A reflective yoga and meditation practice is, I believe a cornerstone to the transformation of the bariatric patient. Being still and in the moment allows us to feel and tune in to the inner dialogue of our selves. In being aware, we are then able to make, as needed, modifications and updates.

The early beginnings of mediation, for me, were in New Hampshire. My parents and grandparents bought a house together when I was five years old. They lived part-time on the upper level of the big green old farmhouse, and we lived downstairs. When they were not in New Hampshire, they lived in a small apartment in New York City. Their two spaces were magical to me—filled with unique treasures, books, pictures, and textures. I would go upstairs when they were gone sometimes and just be alone in their space, feeling their energy.

Above my bedroom was a small room with a severely slanted ceiling line, which made standing impossible the farther into the space one went. The room had a secret hidden door at the lowest part of the ceiling that allowed access to the small attic space. Grandma and Grandpa called this the mediation room.

Every day, they would go to that room and practice bringing the principles of stillness and connectedness to them, skills they learned over the course of years at various retreats around the country. Grandma was always eager to teach me something about meditation, massage, reflexology, or seaweed.

Saturday morning meditation sessions were always a little longer. I wish now that I had taken more advantage of the time we had in my early years, though I guess in revisiting the time and space in my mind, I am reconnecting with them as I find stillness now in my present life.

In the meditation room, the floors were covered, wall to wall with a stack of clean quilted shipping blankets, like the ones movers use to protect furniture. There were three round purple tufted pillows, which were very hard and were used to sit during meditation. Yoga blocks were used to support different challenging yoga poses when it was time for yoga. There were a few books scattered about on the floor, a small statue of the Smiling Buddha, and a window next to a small closet. The chimney on one side offered a beautiful rich earthy feel to the space.

Incense was usually burning somewhere in their apartment; something that gave my father significant irritation, as the scent would, not infrequently, make its way downstairs. To this day, the scent of patchouli brings me immediately back to the Saturday mornings I spent in that space, practicing being quiet and still.

At first stillness is difficult. The mind wants to race and the body does not want to be quiet. With time, patience, and practice, the issues of early meditation wane and meaningful restoration happens.

A truly beautiful side effect of mediation is a feeling of connectedness with the outer world as well as with oneself. Being aware of the small and seemingly inconsequential details that exist in the world allows us to maintain a healthy perspective. The perspective one derives from meditation offers a solid and nearly unshakable foundation on which to

approach the challenges present in day-to-day

activities.

15 Birthday of the Trees

My dear friend was waiting for me. She is well-connected in the local Jewish community, and I feel special being with her. She is smart, articulate, and full of energy! I think I feed off her energy, as I'm confident that given all I've been through today, I would have happily crashed on the couch with a cup of tea and called it a night. Abigail is always pushing me further, and I love that about her.

That night, we were heading to a Tu B'shvat celebration at the local Chabad. My family and I don't attend services there—or anywhere regularly, for that matter. But that night was different. It was the birthday of the trees, and Abigail and I were going to a raw food demonstration/celebration. The air was crisp but not freezing cold like it often is in January. She waited for me in the car, and as I made my rather smooth exit from the house, we greeted each other warmly.

"No coat?" she asked urgently. She was bundled in a down winter parka.

"Nah, if we aren't walking I'm not schlepping a whole coat," I replied.

We drove the three minutes to Chabad, and she miraculously parallel parked her big SUV right at the front entrance to the Chabad temple.

"It sure looks quiet," Abigail said as we pulled up to the old church building. I have always found it jarring that an Orthodox Jewish synagogue is housed in an old church. I must have wrinkled my nose because she added, "It would be like them to cancel and not tell anyone."

I shook my head in disbelief and then checked my negative reaction. I had to remind myself to keep positive thoughts. Letting even one negative thought in can start a spiral that I do not want to bring into my life. We again stepped out into the crisp night air and made our way up the front steps toward the big New England–style brick building with the classic white steeple. Interestingly enough, there is a menorah-like fixture on top of the steeple.

I was not sure what to expect. I thought I remembered that there would be kosher wine and maybe cheese. I was hungry. The breakfast sandwich from Starbucks that I had to eat around eleven hundred was not still with me.

As I recalled my food choices of the day, I was reminded how much I still needed to focus on remembering to eat and making good food choices. I wondered if there would ever be a time when I didn't have to think about food so much. Maybe not. Abigail is very tall, very thin, and often very hungry. I smiled when I had this thought as we reached the top of the granite stairs.

Abigail opened the door, and we walked into the entryway. There were a few young people milling in the breezeway as we hesitantly took our first steps inside. Abigail seemed to feel relaxed and at home there.

A joyous-looking man approached. He was

wearing a plain white linen long-sleeve tunic and had the tzitzit strings hanging out the bottom. He wore a plain black kippah on his head. It was obvious from the wisps of curls that were peeking out from underneath the kippah that he had very curly hair. The curly hair was further evidenced by the very bushy salt-and-pepper gray beard he wore. I learned later that he was the rabbi.

We made our way through the dimly lit open space where high-top tables were set with lovely displays of cheese, grapes, and crackers. The table had a lit candle, which made me smile. In our neutered ultra safe usual lives where battery-operated "candles" reigned king, having real fire was at once thrilling and calming. Abigail and I got our wine and staked out a table. The wine was amazing and the cheese delicious. There were fresh figs, which made me smile. I would never think to buy fresh figs and yet, after that evening, they make a regular appearance when they are in season. Abigail and I made small talk while a clarinet and guitar played soft klezmer music in the background.

After two glasses of wine, I was feeling a delightful easy calm as Abigail and I made our way to the horseshoe-shaped arrangement of tables. Rabbi began to talk to the group—maybe forty-five people—about Tu B'shvat. He had a twinkle in his eyes that gave away what I decided must be a playful spirit. Rabbi held the wine glass carelessly in his hand as he began to talk about the birthday of the trees.

My mind was calm, and I passively took in Rabbi's words. I felt almost as if I was back in the meditation room in Spofford. He was making a metaphor about life and the connectedness of all things with trees and Tu B'shvat. He described five components, which touch me deeply in the moment. I found myself taking notes at a dinner party. Internally, I chuckled. I was still learning. Still searching and, when I am open to it, the universe talks to me.

Out with the Old

First, the rabbi described how old leaves twist off the tree easily and blow away each autumn— meaning that we should let go of the past and let it become the mulch that will nourish something else. In this journey, so much of the work that patients do is related to the twisting off and letting go of the internal dialogue and internal struggles with self-confidence and trust. For me, I was aware of how much I have released out to the universe. The metaphor also related nicely to the release of weight. Dr. V taught his patients about releasing, not losing, weight.

"When we lose things," he would say, "what is the first thing we do? We go looking for them."

Instead, we must change the way our mind connects our process to the physical pounds on the scale. Instead of losing pounds, we release them to the atmosphere. We let the energy go that tied us down, bound us to our own shame and self-loathing, and let it be free. Of course, habits such as self-deprecations and fear can be difficult to break. In time, and with a lot of concerted effort, it is possible to break free the strong prisons we build with our own minds. The trick is to keep the mind free and not let fear or negativity creep back in. I still practice this skill.

Start Small and Let Big Things Develop

The second part of the metaphor is that every

tree starts as a seed; we must start small and let big things develop. The connection to bariatric surgery is again, not difficult to make. There are those who will disagree with this sentiment, who we start small. What is meant by this sentiment is that we must start small because in our smallness, just like a sapling, we are flexible and malleable, able to bear the traumas that change often brings.

In the months immediately following bariatric surgery, I was alive in a way that I'm not sure I ever knew before. My body was changing so rapidly. I was aware of Every. Single. Bite. That went into my body. I ate good food, I exercised, and I changed my internal narrative to a positive monologue. Inevitably, and not unexpectedly, life has a way of happening.

I was finishing making dinner, Jim walked in with a serious face. He is not an overly emotive man, but I could tell he had something important to say.

"Hi, what's up?" I asked.

"Well, remember back a while ago when I told you my window for deployment was going to be opening soon?"

My heart hit the floor. At the time, I had three small children and was alone in Albuquerque, a place I had not entirely adopted as my home. The thought of a deployment to Iraq or Afghanistan was unthinkable. A flurry of emotions filled me: fear, shame, doubt, and disbelief were the first few. I was ashamed to think only of myself in the moment.

Was it not his sworn duty to serve the country—something he had done for nearly ten years faithfully and dutifully? I was afraid that I would not be able to handle my responsibilities at work and at home without him here. Now, after many months, a cross-country move, and a marital separation, I realize that might not have been the easiest thing, but it also sure would not have been the most difficult thing I could have done.

For a number of weeks, and some seriously fretful nights, we discussed what it would be like, how I would manage, and so forth. Jim was prepared to go to the war zone, as directed, but we decided, after a number of conversations, to see if anyone would voluntarily take his slot. Eventually, a few days after offering up the "slot," someone snapped at the opportunity to go to war. Apparently there are people who want to deploy, and to those who are so eager I am eternally thankful.

I realize when I look back at this story that I was scared and rigid, not able to bend and be flexible in the moment. The truth of the matter is, though, I had already given all of my flexibility over to the rest of my life situation (work, kids, family, etc.) and had none left for what felt like an enormous disruption. Eventually, even a willow tree will break in enough wind.

Time and Perseverance Are Required

Third, the rabbi talks about how time and perseverance are two characteristics required by trees and people; we must allow both to grow. We live in a society that values speed and efficiency. Top leaders in business are tasked with finding better ways of guiding operations; professionals are asked to do more with less in most sectors of our society.

Yet, when we go quickly, we can, and often do, miss the opportunity to be fully present. Additionally, when we are hurtling through life at warp speed and something (inevitably) knocks us off our trajectory, the ability to bounce back and get right back up is something many people have difficulty doing. Sometimes, the alteration in the previous trajectory leads to a complete derailment.

We must find a way to develop resilience in our journey, and resilience comes from time and continued practiced perseverance. Also important is the ability to freely and frequently forgive ourselves for the transgressions we believe we have committed against ourselves. Being able to recognize that we are all still working to better ourselves while simultaneously being the very best we can be in any given moment, we can more easily see that we are only capable of being who we are in that moment. By releasing the expectation that we must be "perfect" or "better" or without flaw, we are able to love ourselves a little more deeply, more freely.

The not-so-simple choice to engage in obtaining weight loss surgery, despite many people still assuming that the surgery is an "easy way out," is a very deliberate choice to alter one's individual path. We are choosing to turn our lives upside down. Despite what I thought was a lot of reflection going into the program, I realized during the first week post-op that I was minimally prepared. My body was swollen and sore, and I was unable to take much more than a teaspoon of food/liquid at a time without searing pain (something I avoided like the plague after that one experience with the avocado). I can only imagine those patients who have not gone through the preoperative teaching plan that Dr. V insists on for his patients and without the early exposure my grandparents gave me to being open to the world and accepting of the people who occupy this space in time.

When Is the Best Time?

As we all started to get hungry, the rabbi asked a question. "When is the best time to plant a tree?" He answered his own question, "Forty years ago." He then quickly added, "When is the second-best time to plant a tree? Now!" he shouted.

The meaning to be taken from this line of question and answer is that we should never put off doing something beautiful. The decision to pursue weight loss surgery is not one to be taken lightly. Making the decision to prioritize oneself over others can be challenging, but the rewards are indescribable.

Reaching Upward and Outward

Last, Rabbi talked about the way a tree has a

center trunk and branches that reach out and up from that strong center. The meaning of his last connection is that the stronger the core, the further out and up we can reach, and the sky is the limit! When we are free, and we free ourselves from the ties that bind us, we have no limit.

During the talk, I sat in the banquet chairs next to my dear friend, thinking about how beautiful the metaphor was and how applicable the lessons were to my life right then. My eyes scanned the open space and then settled on the ornate decoration at the front of the temple. The foreign gilded Hebrew script that contrasted starkly with the dark-wood carved fixture were at once calming and perplexing. I wondered about how my own heritage informed who I am.

My mother is Jewish; her mother was Jewish.

My father is Catholic as were both of his parents. As each of my parents tells the story, they wanted to give me a wide experience of faiths and traditions and let me, as an adult, decide what fit best for me. While perhaps nice in theory, the lack of singular direction left me for much of my adult life, feeling lost, divergent, and not connected to any one group.

My dear Catholic family have always been accepting, and while I treasure their inclusion, I have never felt wholly connected because I am neither and both Jewish and/or Catholic. I participate happily in holiday traditions and realized, only once I had left the metro area where they live, how much those traditions and customs influenced who I am today. For example, I am connected to food in terms of celebration and soothing wounds. I have dishes that are prepared in the customary way, which I now realize, must play a smaller part of my new healthier way of being. All the fresh macaroni, pasta, bread and butter, cannoli, and so forth, that once fueled my intersections with the Catholic part of the family now take on a different meaning. The focus on food is something I find I need to actively disengage from. My alternate focus has created some changes in the family dynamic.

Now at family gatherings, I am aware of what I am eating and, more importantly, I am aware that everyone seems to be watching my plate. Of course, this watchful eye comes from a place of love not judgment. I suppose because everyone has a relationship with food, it isn't too difficult to imagine why others would be concerned by what I am eating. Maybe it is as simple as curiosity. For many, as an old friend reminded me, food means a great many things to each of us—far surpassing its foundational function: nutrition.

The emotional connection we humans have to food cannot be overstated. Food is connected to our emotions: stress, fatigue, boredom, happiness, fear, and so forth. Food is used as a drug to try to numb those feelings or to potentiate them. Instead of acknowledging the feeling and actually *feeling* the feeling, we use food to hide, to punish, to celebrate, and to demonstrate our machismo. Try to think of a social gathering where food *is not* part of the event.

The trouble comes when we confuse the consumption of food with the emotion we are trying to hide, potentiate, punish, and so forth. Food is, first and foremost, fuel. When we forget that, and put in our bodies too much fuel or, and this is even more important, the wrong kind of fuel, the body rebels and adds fat and begins disease processes.

Our job is then to remember that each bite is an opportunity to help our bodies function metabolically better or an opportunity to hurt our progress toward balance. Ultimately, we get to choose. We choose which path we are on based on the choices we make. Every day. Every meal. Every time we pass by the fast food, pastry store, deli, et cetera, we are making choices to take back control of one of the very few things we actually have control over.

16 Happy Weight

When starting the journey of weight loss surgery, there really isn't anything that can prepare the individual for the comprehensive life alterations that come. The preoperative teaching in Dr. V's program is amazing and very helpful. To begin a spiritual awakening while simultaneously grabbing hold of one's physical health is a lot to do, though. In fact, even for someone like me who has been exposed to Buddhist teachings and a more inclusive worldview, the total transformation is still breathtaking.

From the simple and somewhat mundane of our physical shape changing to the necessary processing of deep hurts and trauma to the practice of opening up to the world the journey can be exhausting. Add in a partner whose emotional intelligence is not an area of significant strength, and it is little wonder so many relationships have difficulty in the weeks, months, and years following bariatric surgery.

Perhaps the larger issue is that we must remember that our journey does not end. We are continuing to evolve—to change and grow. What was true yesterday, might not be true today. We are all constantly evolving. In that evolution, we must proceed with our eyes open, our hearts open, and our minds open.

Standing in the foyer, I watched the snow falling outside. I could hear the wind whipping through the antique bathroom windows off to one side. I think the curtains were blowing softly. I was standing in that space, thinking about how different my body felt those days. I was not always making the best food choices, and I was frustrated with myself for the transgressions against myself that I had committed. I knew, though, that I must allow forgiveness; instead of being disappointed, I must remember to be gentle with myself as I am gentle with others. I wandered into the living room and plopped on the couch for a much-needed break.

After sitting on the couch in the living room, my nose was cold. I remembered the living room in

Spofford, New Hampshire, where I grew up. I recalled the same feeling in Peabody Massachusetts, where I lived after college. Of course, it didn't seem to penetrate that the reason my nose was cold in the winter had less to do with my nose than it did with passively staying still, watching mindless television in the winter. Because of my many professional and personal obligations, that evening I returned to old habits of sitting still and watching TV. I needed a break, a mental and physical break from the stress and strain of my life.

The time was late, and I needed to get to bed. As I began to drag my weary body off the couch and make my way to the darkened foyer, I realized that my body felt different. I found my hands running down my sides to my waist. It was different—smaller and smoother. Of course my body was different. I'd had bariatric surgery two years before and a cesarean section nine months ago. My body had been through a lot in the last two years. After all, I've released more than a hundred pounds, I have grown a human being, moved across the country, started a new job twice, and begun and completed coursework for a PhD!

I said to a friend recently, "You know how when you have just enough fat, but not too much, it's annoying?"

This friend stared at me blankly. Of course, they had absolutely no idea what I was talking about. This friend was very tall and very slender.

"So, I know you have no idea what I'm talking about," I said.

"No," she replied.

"Well, it's like this: when you are really

overweight, the fat is just part of the experience. There's a lot of it just hanging on. It gets in the way, spills over clothes, wrinkles your pants in all the wrong places, makes wearing nylons impossible, and closing a towel around one's body is laughable. But now, with so much weight released—but not all of it yet—the remaining fat is annoying, in the way."

He continued to stare at me blankly. I was not articulating the idea of "annoying amount of fat" clearly. In the immediate postoperative period, the body is shifting and changing so rapidly. The weight feels like it just flies off! It is difficult to find clothes to fit, partly because the size is changing so rapidly and partly because the mind has not gotten around to being brave enough to try a smaller size and replenish the closet.

For too many years, I refused to buy a larger

size, despite needing one because I didn't want to admit I was that big. Now, after admitting that I needed that size, I wasn't sure I was ready to go back, try again with a now smaller number, and risk the failure of my burgeoning optimism.

The emotional components of being an obese person are so complex and unique to each individual, that describing this phenomenon to others is very difficult, which is why my friend did not quite understand.

Confounding the problem is that right after surgery, there is an impatience to wanting the shape of one's body to shift immediately despite the relative speed that the weight is released. I recall so vividly, Dr. V giving a disclaimer of sorts in the preoperative teaching group that when waking up from surgery, the body shape will be roughly the same size; that we won't immediately be skinny upon waking from the procedure. Of course, as I said, the weight does seem to fly off and there is an adjustment period to wrapping one's head around the new and quickly evolving shape changes, but we live in a society that wants to see results now.

Now, more than one hundred pounds released to the atmosphere, I am noticing how my body moves differently. I am much more apt to get down on the floor and play with my (now) four kids. Now that we live next to the ocean in Massachusetts, I have the energy to go for a walk after dinner on the beach at the end of my street. The release of my weight has not been as fast as that of many other patients, but I am not comparing. One of the important teachings we learn as bariatric patients is that we have to find our "happy weight."

What is a happy weight? Well, it might be a number, it might be a pants size, but the more constructive way to think about this is that it is where we are emotionally happy with our physical size. Everyone will have a different manifestation of the happy weight, and what I am discovering is that the happy weight can (and does) change.

The important part to remember is that negative internal dialogue and hurtful feelings we turn on ourselves must not be part of determining if we are at the happy weight. Too soon we can go back to the old negative emotional habits; when life gets challenging, we can revert to berating ourselves with negative self-talk and self-limiting behaviors.

So, the job for every person, overweight or not, is to find a positive mental space and be happy. Happiness is such an important aspect of our individual and collective journey. Once we decide we are worth it and actively search for it, we inevitably find it. The trick is, to try to prepare so that when happy weight comes, it often brings with it truths that are, at best, uncomfortable.

Having people in one's life who are supportive and loving during this transition is essential—having people with high levels of emotional intelligence who can walk alongside the bariatric patient and support the journey, loving us when we are barely lovable, and helping us reframe our worldview is so incredibly important. For many people, the support person is the chosen life partner. Sometimes he or she is a best friend or family member. Sometimes, as in the case of my business, the person is a wellness support coach.

People seek out my service, my help, when they are struggling with finding happiness and finding their individual purpose and happy weight. They are

seeking someone who has experienced the high peaks

and low valleys and has made it out the other side.

They look for someone to celebrate smaller pants

sizes with or to discuss frustration that the scale isn't

keeping up with their expectations.

17 Labels

Being a bariatric patient, is a label that when applied, still leaves me feeling unsettled. I continue to try to find my place in the world. A label I like less than that of bariatric patient is that of obese person so I accept (begrudgingly) the bariatric patient label. Sort of.

No, when I am most honest, I realize I don't fully accept either label. The obese label I feel much more confident disavowing now, as I am no longer obese, but the bariatric patient label will be harder to release. After all, I will always have been at one point in my life a bariatric patient. Why should that give me grief, though? I decided to take control of my life and to prioritize my needs, my happiness, and my dreams.

When I pause to identify why it is that the label of bariatric patient is unsettling, I discover that the reason has largely to do with my own refusal to accept who I am at the core. Once I am able to fully see myself where there are no lies left, I find peace. The many layers of lies we tell ourselves on any given day are so numerous that to peel them back and truly see who we are is essential to our well-being and our ability to find true happiness.

We all have labels that we apply to ourselves, and there are labels that society places for us. Our job and responsibility is to identify the labels that we have placed on ourselves and let only those that are true stay. For example, I am an intelligent, passionate, loving, kind, and generous person. I give freely my love and support to all who ask for it. I have not always been able to find constructive mechanisms to help me deal with the inevitable struggles that life throws my way, but I will no longer let those opportunities for growth define me.

In fact, I am embracing the opportunity for growth wholeheartedly and am attempting to make positive changes for my individual self and for my family. I have chosen to be the person who grabbed hold of what is truly important and made myself and my own happiness a priority. I have learned new skills and developed new friends and interests. I am creating a new set of labels.

A friend asked me if I wanted to go for a walk with her one day late last summer.

"Sure!" I answered, and then immediately felt nervous. This person, my friend, is a runner and very fit. Did I just agree to walk all the way around the Neck with this person? Would I be able to keep up?

As the evening got closer, I was nervous but determined. I would be just fine. We were to walk around an island that is connected to the mainland. Fancy people, who live in fancy houses, are clustered on the Neck.

So, not only was I going to go exercise with this other fit person, I would be doing so in close proximity to people who, to the outside world, appear surreal. The "Neck People" are beautiful people, fit people. They wear designer workout gear and have garages full of fancy sports cars, and they have boats in the harbor. I know a few people who live there, and they are lovely people, but their day-to-day lives are so different than my own experience that they are, for better or worse, on an unrealistic pedestal.

I pulled into the beach parking lot as the sun was getting low in the sky. My friend and I said hello and started walking out along the causeway. The tide was coming in so the waves on one side of the causeway were large. On the harbor side, boats were everywhere, attached to their moorings. They seem squeezed into the harbor. They were all facing the same angle, as if someone lined them up. The birds flew overhead, lazily getting to their next resting (or fishing) spot.

We always had a lovely time chatting and could literally lose hours in each other's company. I tried to walk quickly and was happily surprised, as I was able to keep pace with her without losing my breath. We chatted about every possible topic, and we were completely enjoying our time together. Somehow, I mentioned what a big step it was for me to be doing this kind of activity.

"Why?" my friend asked, completely puzzled.

"Well, I've never considered myself an "active" person," I replied.

"Really? But I see you all the time now at the gym and walking and playing with the kids," she said.

"Well, yes. I suppose you are right. But before the surgery, I would have *never* considered going for a walk/jog with someone. I would have never imagined I would be able to even make it around the Neck, let alone on display with a friend! In fact, I have come out to the Neck so many times to rest and recover, to think, to process an idea or situation countless times. But I've done so in my car. I don't think in all the years I've lived in this area I have *ever* walked around the Neck."

As I said those words, I realized that I had created a new label for myself. I was now someone who could (and did) exercise for a girls' afternoon/evening out. Opportunities now existed for me to consider going for a run on the beach, or doing stand-up paddle boarding. I could now stop limiting my life because I was physically not able and start doing whatever I *wanted* to do and not just the things I thought I *could* do.

I had been limiting myself by thinking that there was no way I could have accomplished the three-mile walk around the Neck. The distance felt so intimidating because I had only ever done it in my car. As we walked, talked, and enjoyed each other's company, I showed myself that it was achievable.

I have since walked the Neck a number of times, each time noticing a new detail or experiencing the streets with a new excitement. I am an active person who can exercise *with* people and enjoy myself in the process!

My narrative continues to evolve. My sights are now set on Mt. Kilimanjaro in Africa. I will climb that mountain in the summer of 2017 with a group. I have purchased the boots; I have begun to practice hiking. I am now a person who will climb tall mountains!

18 Reality

Reality is perception. Our day-to-day experiences are influenced solely by our perceptions, our history, and our understanding. I am sitting in my office cube, freezing as the bright sun pours through the window behind me. In this moment, I become aware that the reality of the sunshine is quite disparate from the way that I feel at the moment; the sun shines and I freeze.

Rachel West

This is such a typical New England sensation. There are days in the winter that are so beautiful with bright blue skies, and even brighter sunshine, but the moment I stick my nose outside, I am immediately reminded that it is winter, and therefore I should stay as far away from the outside as humanly possible without many layers on my shrinking body!

I believe that we can shape who we are and what we want in how we think, what we say, how we act, and with whom we associate. We are a summation of our experiences and our collective memory of our experiences. Following bariatric surgery, the scope of change that patients experience is profound and causes a dynamic and sometimes explosive shift. Everything changes.

For example, as I got dressed one morning I put on the lanyard that holds the identification badge I

172

use to open doors. I caught a glimpse of myself in the mirror as I walked by. I noticed the badge freely hanging as I walked by. No longer does the badge rest on my abdomen. No longer is it lost in folds somewhere. Swaying side to side, my badge has free motion in the universe. If only I would allow my mind to be that free.

Just the fact that I noticed myself in the mirror represents a change. How many mirrors have I hurried by so that I didn't have to see myself? How many plate glass windows never saw a glance because I didn't want to see my reflection? Until very recently, there were no mirrors in my home. The people who lived in the house before my family, took the mirrors off the walls for some reason before they left. I had to buy a small mirror just so I could fix my hair in the morning.

Now, I have a full length mirror in the bedroom, and I find that I want to see how the entire outfit works in the morning. I want to change how my mind holds the vision of me with a new narrative. I am reshaping my reality.

The beauty of realizing that we are the masters of our own reality comes in knowing that if true, anything is possible. Sometimes knowing that anything is possible is scary, and full transcendence has not quite become my reality; the mirror is propped up on the floor covered by a spare chair and a pile of clothes. I have made the situation so that I still have to work to see my true self.

If we accept the belief that we control very little beyond our reaction to the world around us, and we do not control our feelings or our thoughts, as the psychologists say, how can we find peace with our new selves? We practice. We practice embracing the world for what it is and trying to be open to the messages we receive.

Reading and writing about the practice of spiritual enlightenment and self-discovery are two very important habits for any new bariatric patient. Because the procedure is what it is—a surgical adjuvant to emotional growth and change—becoming aware of how to find our truest selves is critically important.

What is the true self? The true self is the self that lies at the bottom, where no lies are left. By continuing to reshape the internal narrative along with the external picture of who we are—truly—we are able to engage in a more emotionally healthy way.

Transformations

In the journey of significant weight loss and becoming an adult, major transformations are inevitable. Now, a few years' post-op and an equally long reflective period, I am sure that the old me has died. But is she really gone? Tomorrow would mark my grandmother's birthday—the grandmother whose sharp words, said with love, started this entire process.

When I think back now, I realize that even though she is gone from my day-to-day life, she is still here. She still shapes who I am becoming. Is the same true for the old me? Is she really gone? There are times when my life is still consumed with self-doubt and shame; two attributes of my former self. What is it that keeps them here?

I was working at a large private university in Boston, teaching undergraduate nursing students. The class sizes were huge: 120 students in each section. The school utilized a co-teaching structure, and so there were always two professors in each classroom environment. My thoughts about the disservice such large class sizes have on metacognition and the development of safe, proficient, high-quality nurses is a topic for another book. Suffice to say, there is a lot of running from place to place to meet all the needs of the students.

On one rainy day, my co-teacher and I were hurrying to get to class. It was test day, and we wanted to get sort of organized before giving one of the high-stakes exams to our group of *very* nervous nursing students. Somehow, we left later than we intended, and our preparation time was shrinking quickly as we made our way into the main campus building.

The line for the elevator to the third floor was very long and the elevators were notoriously slow. I am not sure what possessed me, but I said to my very petite ex-army officer nurse co-teacher, "let's just take the stairs."

Immediately after the words passed my lips, dread filled me. What did I just suggest? Sprint up three flights of stairs? *WITH* another woman? I was sure I must have lost my mind. How on earth would I ever be able to keep my breath under control? There was no way, in my mind, that I would be fit enough to get up the stairs unscathed.

We approached the stairs and a voice from deep inside me offered up a rather positive thought. I heard my inner voice tell my anxious self: You aren't that person anymore. You can do this. You might not be as fit as she is, but you will make it up three flights of stairs!

While we climbed, I noticed that I was not terribly out of breath. The flights of stairs were long and I started getting dizzy from all of the turning around and around on the split stairs, but I was generally fine. When we got to the top, I smiled. My colleague caught me. I felt obliged to explain some of what I was feeling.

"I don't think I ever would have even attempted a three-flight climb with another person before. I guess I really am a new person."

She didn't quite understand but after I told her the super short version of bariatric surgery a few years prior and large weight loss, she seemed to sort of get the magnitude of the success I was feeling.

The truth is, people who have not struggled

with weight like obese people have do not really understand the limits we place on ourselves. I had been consciously and unconsciously limiting my activities because I was afraid I would be out of breath or that someone might judge me. In reality, people are going to judge, but their judgment does not need to be any concern of mine. I was reminded later, as I walked up and down the auditorium rows proctoring the test, of a quote that is quite applicable: other people's opinions of me are none of my business.

That test day was a turning point for me. I felt and accepted the lessons from that experience. I learned to push myself some out of my "comfort zone" because that zone has, too often, been limited by distorted thoughts. I learned to let other people judge how they will and not give those judgments another thought! Most of the time, I can remember to let go of other people's perceptions. In the moments I feel the opinions of others coming in, I stop the thought train and let it float away and remember that their opinion of me is none of my business.

In order to move forward, along the path of our own individual journey in weight loss, we must let go of the past and be free. We must allow the past to die and clear the way for the present. In doing so, we are able to process what is immediately in front of us and go about the world attaining self-actualization.

Self-actualization is a term that I have always thought is reserved for some unattainable state of being. I have since studied Maslow several times in my educational career, and I even teach some of the concepts in my classes. It was not until very recently that I became fully aware of what it means to reach (and sustain) self-actualization.

Being self-actualized can be described in five interconnected themes. First, being self-actualized means that the individual is aware of the real world around him or her. Individuals are accepting of reality and have realistic perceptions of themselves and the world.

Additionally, people who are self-actualized are focused on problems, including helping others and finding solutions to problems. Self-actualized people are spontaneous and are often described as unconventional people who value independence, privacy, and solitude to allow for personal introspection as they reach their full potential. Lastly, people who are self-actualized see the world around them as awe-inspiring and often experience moments of intense joy and wonder.

I have sought more information about how to translate and relate to one of the founding fathers of modern psychology, Abraham Maslow. His hierarchy of needs is a description of building blocks for personal fulfillment. I realize, in my search, that I am a person who is reaching for self-actualization, a fact that surprises me and fills me with joy and satisfaction. I am continuously amazed at how the effect of a few people, including my grandmother and a dear friend, can so profoundly impact how I go about my day-to-day activities. I am introspective and aware of the reality of the world around me.

Grandma used to use the phrase "deal with reality" so much that for a while, my mother and I were traumatized by the word "reality." We would both recoil whenever Grandma would remind us that we were straying off course. Of course, I know now that dealing with reality means being present, aware,

and in awe of the world around me. I am, every day,

still hoping to learn something new and in the process

living my true purpose.

19 Shame

Shame and self-doubt are two emotions that are absolutely disparate from self-actualization. However, these two emotions are still present in my life as I continue to work out the nuances of the new "me." The old me is dead, as I said before. She was negative and afraid, punishing and severe, sad and lonely. The truth is I still feel all those emotions. The difference now is that when I notice I am feeling them, I turn inward to determine the true cause—the reality—so that I can learn what lesson I need from it and be able to move on.

As my marriage started to truly fall apart, I became much more introspective. I sought out friends to confide in and share experiences with. I began to make another life, one where I was free to be the version of myself I felt was hiding for so long. I joined a mahjong group, and I began to journal extensively and to write this book. I wanted to know and learn what it was that drove me to where I was in the present moment.

Interestingly, the process of turning in—while helpful in the short run—is not all that helpful in the longer timeframe of the rest of my many days. The rituals we make and keep are what drive us to our goals. We are what we do.

A secret Internet group has hundreds of

members who are affiliated with Dr. V and/or his clinic. The online atmosphere, attitude, and general vibe are some of the most positive anywhere on the Internet. The live sessions are equally excellent but are reserved for current local patients—which I am not.

The online community of bariatric patients supported by Dr. V is so special. Participants ask questions, give support, post transformation pictures, provide encouragement, and share positive and uplifting quotes and images. Negativity is simply not tolerated. There are few places where people can be totally honest and discuss obesity-related issues freely, without fear of judgment, and this is one of them.

After we began the process of separation, I felt a noticeable sting whenever I would go to the online group. I felt hurt and sadness instead of comfort and joy when visiting and checking in with other patients. My first instinct was to turn inward; run away. I wrote to my fellow sleeve family, and prepared to say good-bye for a while.

Interestingly, but not surprisingly, in less than forty-eight hours, I was feeling so rotten, disconnected, and alone. I had separated from the safe online space where I had been so active for so long, and I began to grieve. By turning inward, I realized I was running away, retreating to safety. But instead of feeling better, I felt much worse. What had this online group full of people I largely had never met really meant to me? What was it about them that was so special?

What I have determined is that the members of the group are all actively dedicated to purposefully being positive and supportive of one another. Where else in our lives do we experience such unconditional love? By celebrating successes and sharing my thoughts in the group, I believe that I have something meaningful to contribute, and that makes me feel so good.

It still stings to be there. They are, and it is nowhere near their fault, an ever-present reminder of the transformation that helped me remember and uncover who I am today. While I still have some work to do to accept the label of bariatric patient (we are ALL flawed, remember), being there, in that group helps.

I am still hurting, but I am convinced that one of the best places to go is to the group, my unconditionally loving "family." No one knows what path we are all walking. Not our providers or our partners. The patients and the patients alone understand the emotional toll this kind of awakening brings. Why would I deny myself the salve their support brings?

So I decided to tell them all of this and rejoin the positive and uplifting community of bariatric patients. They embraced me with open and loving arms. Of course they did. They know what a challenge and opportunity this journey can be. I am forever grateful for their kind generosity during my pain.

20 Attachment

Buddhist teachings are interwoven in the bariatric program where I had my procedure. Dr. V is not trying to create a center of Buddhists; he says he is not Buddhist. But many of the principles that Buddha taught are, as one becomes aware, part of the program. One that is of particular interest in my journey and the resulting dissolution of my marriage is the theory of attachment. There are many excellent resources out there about the theory of attachment in Buddhism, and they may be of interest for further study. I will share what I know.

Basically, attachment, as I understand the principle, means that when people have a desire for something, they see that something as being outside of themselves. So, for people to have attachment, they have to have something to crave, and then the active pursuit of that "thing" is the attachment. Attachment requires self-reference, the ability to see ourselves as separate and apart from what we desire, which is contradictory to basic Buddhist teachings.

I wonder though, don't we have a responsibility to ourselves? Don't we need to have a responsibility to others, even though we are all connected? I have been thinking a lot about attachment and what that means. I have come to understand that the absolute worst deceptions we have are those we play on ourselves.

Of course, by seeing the things we "want" as being outside of ourselves and then chasing after people, things, feelings, and so forth (the attachment), we are creating a deception of reality. Not only does chasing, sometimes referred to as thirst in Buddhist teachings, result in deceptions of reality, it creates attachments. Attachments can be for things, material possessions, money, et cetera, and can be nonmaterial things like anxiety in love.

Letting go of the pain of our deceptions by letting go of the craving to capture, and thus control the deception, will help us to access the light within us. The light will guide us, and peace will surround our souls.

We are nothing but energy. Energy, we know

from the study of physics (yet, something I have

miraculously managed to avoid in my long

educational career), cannot be created or destroyed.

So, our human work is to somehow simultaneously

hold and let go; to connect to the universe and let the

universe guide us.

Bariatric patients have a unique opportunity

to practice the Buddhist principle of nonattachment

then as we attempt to not see ourselves as distinct and

separate but unified with the universe and as

inextricably linked to one another. Therefore, in order

to practice this philosophy, we must be willing to let

go completely. I am convinced after what feels like a

long time practicing, the integration of the

nonattachment paradigm will take much more

practice.

In fact, it is the application of nonattachment

principles that helped me rejoin the online community. We belong to each other. We support the struggles others are experiencing and we celebrate together the many victories. There are times though, that the process of letting go is very difficult. Of course, the saying goes that when we are too busy to meditate for ten minutes, we should meditate for twenty. I think a similar principle is at work with practicing nonattachment. The more I practice, the better I will become at the outcomes I desire—that I know are good.

21 High Tide

I have come to this place countless times to look out over the coastal islands and the harbor. Sometimes the mouth of the harbor is busy with lobster boats, pleasure boats, and sailboats. Other times, like today, the harbor is quiet. The sun is shining brightly and the blue of the sky pops over the landscape. It is still too early for leaves to be out on trees or for fishing boats to be in the harbor. A few more days like today with good weather though, and I think to myself that we will start seeing boats pop up on the moorings soon, waiting to be used and loved.

I have lived on the North Shore of Boston for twelve of the last twenty years. I moved out of my childhood home to come here. I attended college, got my first apartment, paid my first bills, and had my heart broken for the first time all here on the North Shore. There are few other places where I feel quite so grounded; where I have so much cogent history.

The rounded soft-brown-colored center column holds the enclosed stairwell of the lighthouse and is then surrounded by steel scaffold-looking bars. The structure is capped by a rust-smeared black light housing. The bright green light shines brightly in the evening hours but now, as it is daytime, the light is not shining.

Just over the rocky ledge, the ocean laps at

the jagged shore. There are two or three seagulls dotting the surface of the blue-green waves. No one is here but me and my thoughts this sunny morning. The waves are quiet today unlike my mind. I am thinking about the life I have led, the life I am leading, and the life that I want. I find that I have more questions than answers, and that unnerves me.

I think about what it might be like to leave this area again. I have had to leave this area before when I was first married. Jim was an officer in the air force and so was stationed all around the country. I cried and cried when I realized that we would, in fact, have to leave Massachusetts. Now, as I have taken a big step in my professional career—to chase a job that is at once scary and exciting across the country—I am reminded of the loathing, sinking feelings I had before when I think about maybe having to leave again.

The lighthouse, as we can probably easily agree is a grounding place; it is the thing that mariners use to guide them safely along the otherwise treacherous coastline. Perhaps one reason that I feel so grounded here is related to that ingrained imagery, or perhaps it is because I have come to this parking lot so many times to find my own footing.

I have come here for years to look out over the harbor, to the harbor islands, and beyond to the horizon on sunny days and cold dark nights. I have come when I am content and when sad. My kids have played on the rock formations, and I have sat happily on the benches that dot the open space.

Today, a big black-and-white seagull lifts off from the tiny waves it has been riding and soars in the bright blue sky up toward the top of the lighthouse. I am brought back to my mind, to my dreams where I see my goals taking me.

Perhaps the greatest gift bariatric surgery has given me is the gift to continue to reevaluate my goals, to keep imagining bigger goals and feeling able to reach for them. I still fear failure, but now I am much more willing to spread my wings and imagine a different path.

We have spent our lives trying to make the best decisions we can in the moments we have. As a result of our life experiences, some of us have developed decision-making and coping skills that are flawed and lead us to consume too many unhealthy foods. When life throws us a curveball, we seek food for solace. When we feel happy, we celebrate with a cupcake. When we are stressed, we reach for our so-called comfort food.

The inevitable self-loathing shame and

negative narrative follows. We know better than to reward ourselves with food, and yet we do it because we have not spent the time to think about another way. Until now.

Now, knowing that those coping mechanisms are not healthy emotionally and physically, we can make adjustments and choose a new path. Making new skills that stick in the moment when we are tested takes time and patience. I have the time, and I am building the patience.

22 Relationships

I come to the end of a long path. I wait. I listen and hear the waves, the birds, and the buzz of spring's first bugs. I let my eyes stretch out to the open sea. Seagulls soar and plummet to the waves, hoping to catch a clam or a fish, perhaps. The waves are strong today but not overpowering. It seems as though the ocean means business—as though today it will not be passive.

Today, the ocean and I, we are the same—

directed, not passive. I notice the sparkle of the sun dance along the mini peaks of the vast open space and think to myself that it looks like a trillion little mirrors dancing on the surface. This thought makes me smile, which is, unfortunately, a rare occurrence these days.

I am standing, waiting, observing. I can feel the mounting pain of what is coming. I know it was I who initiated pain, through the separation, for so many, and remembering that tears at my heart. I am a healer, not the one who inflicts the pain. I feel my own saltwater tears bubble up in my eyes and my throat begin to swell. I take a deep breath and let the optimist in me bring calming thoughts up to the surface: the pain that is here now will heal in time. We will all become stronger. I have hope for that.

I try to remember that I must not let negativity in; that by letting the negative in, I am weakened by it. Negativity is like an incoming wave; it gets bigger and bigger and bigger until it crests and crashes, obliterating everything in its wake.

The negative thoughts will grow to crowd out the positive, and I cannot let that happen. I have worked too hard and fought too long, to let negative thoughts rule my mind and life.

"It is too warm for March," I hear myself think aloud. The tide is coming in and I can tell I have been standing here for a while, as the rock I had been watching is now completely covered by the water. The smell of the fresh salt air invigorates me. I begin to walk back toward home. Usually, the water calms my mind and soothes my spirit. Today though, I am not calmed. I am hurt and feeling very alone. The tide is coming in, and with it will come more pain. I know this and try to brace myself for the impact.

When the inevitable impact comes, I am bowled over. Never in my wildest dreams did I ever envision myself inflicting as much pain and sadness as I did when I ended my nearly ten-year marriage. I knew it was the right decision in the moment. I needed a partner who my chosen partner could not be. I had, for the bulk of our marriage, not looked clearly at the real situation, the real circumstances, or my real needs and desires. Instead, I saw only what I wanted to see that would satisfy my vision of good and right. I made decisions about the reality I wanted, not the reality I had.

I wanted stability, and I found it. I held strongly to stability—so strongly that I strangled out the other aspects of myself that I needed so desperately to express, but which I had suppressed. Those desires and needs were kept hidden underneath my weight. Then, as the weight left and my true self reappeared, I saw just how much of my life and my choices were not congruent with what I really needed and really wanted.

I tried asking for help. We sought counseling individually and together. I meditated and found my inner kindness. We tried more date nights, time out, and desperately tried to reconnect with each other. I lowered my expectations, and I ignored the pain. The truly horrible part of the process was that in asking for separation, I felt like I was asking for elective cosmetic surgery for something so contextually ridiculous that I could scarcely be taken seriously.

I was asking to begin a painful process that would affect many people because I was not having my needs met. There was no abuse, no horrible living situation, nothing terrible to report or point out to those who asked the truly horrendous "what happened?" questions. I had to justify why I wanted more.

Because he and I had, over the years, considered ending the marriage a number of times, this time I felt I had to be sure that I was sure; I was and I am. I grieved losing a companion. I grieved losing the idea of the life we could have had someday. I grieved the impact this would have on my kids as a result of my choice to put myself and my needs first. I hoped that in time they would see that I was showing them how to stand up for themselves, to love themselves, and to make sure they make the best decisions they can for themselves. Of course, in the moment it was rather traumatic.

The process of separation, I am so grateful, has been challenging but amiable. We are still in the house together, but now my expectations have changed. How much of our lives would be spent in a happier place if we could learn to mitigate our expectations and let people be who they really are? Of course, as individuals, we need to check in with ourselves to determine if we know who our true selves really are before making decisions. Once our true selves are brought to the forefront, we can make decisions that will not in time turn to regret.

Relationships with other people have changed after bariatric surgery, too. I was, for a long time, hesitant to tell people that I had the surgery because of the stereotypes surrounding the procedure. But for those people I care to have the discussion with, to clear up misconceptions, to facilitate understanding, I have discovered a much deeper and more meaningful relationship. Everyone who has been let into the circle has been supportive and loving; for that, I know I am blessed.

The journey through bariatric surgery is one that has been for me accompanied by a spiritual awakening. I am now more tuned in to the world around me and more aware of the fragility of life and the absolute necessity for us all to remember that we belong to one another.

The time we have on this earth is short; we must remove our masks and live according to the rules of our truest selves. Keep evolving, keep searching, and choose happiness.

Be in the moment. After all, the moments are all we have. And this one is already gone.

Rachel West

About the Author

Rachel West is a nurse, mother of four small children, and the owner of Driftwood Wellness Group. Driftwood Wellness Group is a consulting company, providing support coaching to those engaged in bariatric surgical and nonsurgical weight loss. The company also offers workshops as well as individual coaching sessions to small and large local and international audiences. She has practiced nursing for the last sixteen years in a variety of settings including intensive care, hospice, administration, and most recently, academics. She is both a teacher and a student, grateful for the opportunity to share knowledge and receive insights from wherever they may come.

Check out Rachel's website:
www.driftwoodwellnessgroup.com

Follow Rachel on Facebook and Twitter:
@driftwoodwellnessgroup

Rachel West

Big Changes from a Small Stomach

www.ingramcontent.com/pod-product-compliance
Lightning Source LLC
Chambersburg PA
CBHW052128270326
41930CB00012B/2800